GARLAND STUDIES ON THE ELDERLY IN AMERICA

edited by
STUART BRUCHEY
University of Maine

A GARLAND SERIES

COHESIVENESS AND COHERENCE

RELIGION AND THE HEALTH OF THE ELDERLY

ELLEN L. IDLER

GARLAND PUBLISHING, INC.
NEW YORK & LONDON / 1994

Library of Congress Cataloging-in-Publication Data

Idler, Ellen L.
    Cohesiveness and coherence : religion and the health of the elderly /
Ellen L. Idler.
        p.   cm. — (Garland studies on the elderly in America)
    Includes bibliographical references (p. xxx-xxx) and indexes.
    ISBN 0-8153-1632-1 (alk. paper)
    1. Aged—United States—Religious life—Case studies.   2. Aged—
United States—Health and hygiene—Case studies.   3. Health—
Religious aspects—Case studies.   I. Title. II. Series.
BL625.4.I35   1994
200'.84'6—dc20   93-48507
                                                                            CIP

Printed on acid-free, 250-year-life paper
Manufactured in the United States of America

Table of Contents

List of Tables

List of Figures

Preface

In the very big and interdisciplinary field of the social scientific study of human aging, there has been extremely little attention paid to the religious beliefs and practices of elderly people. This is a surprising blind spot when you consider the importance of religion to many great classical theorists in social science, among them Emile Durkheim and Max Weber, William James and Gordon Allport.

This study, originally a dissertation in sociology at Yale University, was begun in the excitement of the then very new findings that connections to social networks appeared to protect individuals against mortality. Studies of large, population-based samples in Alameda County, California, Tecumseh County, Michigan, and Evans County, Georgia, were consistently showing that individuals with social ties to family, friends, community groups, and churches or synagogues had lower risks of mortality than those who did not. These late twentieth-century findings took a form that was surprisingly similar to Durkheim's early twentieth findings that social life protected people from suicide. Religion had played an important role in Durkheim's study of the risk of suicide, and it also appeared to protect people from mortality from all causes in the later studies. But few studies particularly focused on religion and health followed the broad social network studies.

One of the problems in studying religion and health in surveys is that the data on religious involvement are often limited to a single question on the frequency of attendance at religious services. This is a problem, of course, especially for studies of elderly populations, where poor health may prevent attendance at services. I recall reading a questionnaire used in a survey pretest where the question "How often do you attend religious services?" was coded "Never." In the margin, though, the interviewer had written "but priest comes to house once a week." In such a survey, we would not be surprised to see that attendance at religious services was associated with better health among the respondents, but we would be doing little but using religion as a crude proxy for physical functioning.

The data used in the study reported in this monograph come from the Yale University site of the National Institute on Aging's Established Populations for the Epidemiologic Study of the Elderly, a longitudinal study of the health and well-being of a population sample of New Haven elderly. From the point of view of the study of religion and health, the great virtue of these data is that they contain questions not only about the public, social aspects of religious practice, but also about the individual's private religious feelings and beliefs, attitudes which would not be dependent on physical ability or health. In addition, the data contain measures of chronic illness, functional ability, depression symptoms, and overall ratings of health given by the individual respondents. The sample is large and representative of the community, and the response rates were very high. All in all, it is an ideal set of data for testing the hypothesis that religious involvement promotes well-being in elderly individuals.

The theoretical perspective of the study is that religious involvement of all kinds does promote physical and mental health among elderly people, for several reasons. For one thing, people in religious groups are known to have better health practices and to live more moderate lifestyles with respect to cigarette smoking, alcohol consumption, and sexual activities. The reduction in these known risk factors would alone lead to better health levels. Moreover, the accumulation of lifelong practices could be expected to produce the most dramatic differences among elderly cohorts. The *health behavior hypothesis* says that the effect of religious involvement on health is due simply to the better health practices of the more religious elderly.

Beyond this, the religious institution offers the benefits of social ties with others in one's community. Durkheim's theory was that religious groups, some perhaps better than others, would reduce the risk of suicide in their members by regulating behavior and by promoting feelings of belonging or social integration. We might expect to see enhanced differences between religious and nonreligious elderly here too. The religious group provides a stable source of intergenerational social contact for elderly people which may balance the losses of same-age friends and siblings. Religious groups traditionally offer tangible material and emotional support to those in need. They also offer opportunities for serving others in a social role that cannot be lost because of bereavement or retirement. This, in a word, is *the cohesiveness hypothesis*, that religion provides the elderly person with a protective social niche, a place of belonging and a source of support. The cohesiveness hypothesis most closely matches the Durkheimian theoretical basis of the social network/social support studies of mortality.

The coherence hypothesis takes a cognitive approach to the problem of religion and health. Max Weber, in *The Sociology of Religion*, describes religious revelation as providing "coherent meaning" for "both social and cosmic events." Perhaps even more important than their social support functions, religious groups are characterized by their shared beliefs about the sacred, about ethical principles for guiding behavior, and about the meaning of human life and death. Religious beliefs may for some elderly people promote a lifelong sense of meaning and purpose and a comforting belief in an afterlife. What makes the cognitive approach so important is that these beliefs need not be diminished by the illnesses or disabilities which prevent attendance at religious services, indeed they may be enhanced by them. There are reasons for thinking that coherent belief systems might be of particular benefit to the health and well-being of elderly people, and the importance of measuring both private and public forms of religious involvement becomes especially clear.

A fourth hypothesis takes the view that the resources of the religious group will come into play primarily in the presence of crisis. In the social support literature, this view has become known as the buffering, or stress-buffering hypothesis. Providing meaning in times of acute suffering is one of the singular functions of religion, a manifest and not a latent one. The range of health problems available in the data offered an opportunity to test the idea that religious involvement would moderate the consequences of poor health. *The theodicy hypothesis*, then, proposes that respondents will respond to chronic illnesses and functional disability with fewer depressive symptoms and poor self-assessments of health when they have access to religious interpretations of their troubles, or to the emotional support of the religious congregation.

The findings of the analyses reported here strongly support the hypothesis that religious involvement will be associated with better health, in particular with fewer chronic conditions, better physical functioning, fewer symptoms of depression, and better subjective ratings of health. The support for the explanatory hypotheses was mixed; most interesting were a number of significant interactions which indicated support for the theodicy hypothesis. The findings overall tended to be stronger for women than for men, and the effect of public religious involvement was generally greater than the effect of private beliefs.

A portion of the findings reported in this monograph were published in the journal *Social Forces* (Idler, 1987). The weakness of the findings, from a methodological point of view, was that they are based on data from 1982 only. In other words, the data were cross-sectional, making causal interpretations difficult since religious involvement and health status were measured at the same time. This would be a problem with any research on social factors in health because poor health levels would themselves tend to diminish the size and frequency of contact with social networks. The individuals remaining in the large social networks would be *selected* for their health status, and any finding of an association between the two could be as much a result of this selection as it is a causal relationship.

The approach taken to address the problem of selection was to arrange the health status outcome measures in a hierarchy beginning with medically-diagnosed conditions and ending with the subjective ratings of health status, and to include each of the more objective measures in the multivariate analysis of the more subjective indicators of health status. This allows a comparison of, for example, the depression symptoms of the more religious with the less religious elderly at any given level of chronic illness and disability. There was reason to believe that the patterns of better health and greater religious involvement were not entirely due to selection, but with cross-sectional data, one couldn't be sure.

So several years of follow-up later, Stanislav Kasl and I did a longitudinal analysis of the same sample and were very pleased to obtain almost exactly the same findings as the cross-sectional analysis had shown. These findings were published in the *American Journal of Sociology* (Idler and Kasl, 1992). Having longitudinal data meant that we were looking at the effect of religious involvement (in 1982) on *changes* in health status that occurred in the period following 1982, when the effects of selection were removed. In this article we also showed that Christians and Jews tended to die less frequently in the month before their own group's religious holidays, another important finding showing the effect of religious involvement on health status. All in all, the later findings provide strong validation for the findings of the early study, and it might easily not have happened that way.

Despite having been written some years ago, then, the following study remains one of the very few on the subject of religion and the health of the elderly. The combination of good data on health status with any measures of religious involvement at all remains a rarity in population samples, and follow-up data are even more unusual. The biggest contribution the following work could make is to show, not only that the empirical relationship between religious involvement and well-being is substantial, but that it presents a truly engaging set of intellectual questions.

For these data I am extremely grateful to the respondents, investigators, and staff of the New Haven EPESE site, the Yale Health and Aging Project. Lisa Berkman and Adrian Ostfeld, Co-Principal Investigators of the project gave me permission to use the data, and Linda Leo graciously made it available. Lisa Berkman, Blair Wheaton, and Jerome Myers pushed me to link the analytical and the conceptual and set high standards for me with their own work. Stan Kasl is responsible for having the questions about religion in the survey in the first place, and it has been a pleasure to collaborate with him on the later work. During the period of writing I was supported by a National Institute of Mental Health Predoctoral Traineeship in the Department of Sociology at Yale University, and by a Woodrow Wilson Foundation Charlotte Newcombe Dissertation Fellowship. All have given me more than I have given them and I am profoundly grateful; the failings of the work are entirely my own.

New Brunswick, New Jersey   E.I.
August 1993

References

Idler, Ellen L. "Religious Involvement and the Health of the Elderly: Some Hypotheses and an Initial Test" *Social Forces* 66(1987):226-38.

Idler, Ellen L. and Stanislav Kasl. "Religion, Disability, Depression, and the Timing of Death" *American Journal of Sociology* 97(1992):1052-79.

Introduction

If any man is favored with long life, it is God that has
lengthened his days. They who walk in the way of
righteousness, shall be honored with living to Old Age,
when the wicked shall have their days shortened, which
indeed many times happen to be so, yet not always.

Increase Mather (1716)

The connection between religion and longevity was an evident
one to the eighteenth century New England mind. In a culture where
little escaped religious interpretation, it should not be surprising that,
given the high infant mortality rate, the fairly rare event of living to
middle and old age occasioned religious comment. Moreover, in
Calvinist New England, growing old was one of the most obvious signs
of grace, (though not a certain one, as Increase Mather notes, only the
righteous aged could be *certain* of election). Nevertheless, old men
were thought to look like God; or as Mather wrote in the sermon, "The
Dignity and Duty of Aged Servants," "There is something of the Image
of God in age." The New England theocracy venerated its old men,
who were believed to have "a peculiar acquaintance with the Lord
Jesus" (Cotton Mather, 1690). The Puritans did not revere all of their
elderly citizens, it must be said; women and the aged poor were not
accorded the same veneration as elder clergy. Nevertheless it was the
elderly, even if only a small group of elderly men, who dominated the
society's institutions. They were given the best seats in church; the
term Elders was no euphemism. And they held nearly complete
political as well as ecclesiastical power. The wisdom they had was that
of the greatest accumulation of experience: if they were thought to be
closer to the next world, they were also closer to the past. They were,
in a very broad sense, the bearers of their culture.

The religious beliefs of eighteenth century New England are
hardly more peculiar to the twentieth century mind than their beliefs
about the aged. This revolution in age relations and attitudes toward the
elderly has been recently of great interest to social historians (Fischer,
1978; Achenbaum, 1978) but that is not at issue here.   It is the very

peculiarity of the idea that there is any connection at all between religion and the health of the elderly that concerns me. What was a perfectly obvious relationship to seventeenth, eighteenth, and early nineteenth century Americans has become a questionable, not-much-thought-about epidemiological hypothesis.

It is because the subject of religion and health has not been much thought about that this study will be highly interdisciplinary in perspective. If there were an established body of research on religion and health in psychosocial epidemiology, the sociology or psychology or anthropology of religion, or social gerontology, it would be possible to narrow its focus more. But in a field with little theory or research, the range of relevant work is as broad as it is thin. In that sense, then, this is an exploratory study, in which a broad range of theoretical approaches and hypotheses are explored. They will be tested on data from the Yale University Health and Aging Project, a major survey of the physical health and social environment of the elderly currently under way in New Haven, Connecticut. The following analyses present results from the baseline interviews, conducted in 1982. Thus it is also an exploratory study in the sense that no very conclusive answers can be reached, given the tentativeness of the hypotheses and cross-sectional nature of the data.

Chapters I and II each examine one aspect of the complex relationship of religion and the health status of the elderly. In Chapter I the basic argument is made for the study's overall hypothesis that there will be a positive association between religious participation and health, specifically that higher levels of both public and private religious involvement will be related to better subjective health and functional ability, and to fewer chronic illnesses and feelings of depression. Three intervening, explanatory hypotheses are then advanced which may account for some or all of the positive relationship between religious involvement and health: a health behavior hypothesis, that focuses on the effects of religious participation at the physiological level; a social cohesiveness hypothesis, which makes its argument at the level of social relationships; and a sense of coherence hypothesis which is primarily cognitive in orientation. More specifically, the health behavior hypothesis proposes that religious participation acts primarily by promoting certain health habits or activities that reduce known risk factors such as smoking or drinking. The social cohesiveness or social integration hypothesis argues along Durkheimian lines that religious participation offers the still-mysterious health benefits of social networks and social support. Finally, the coherence hypothesis takes the Weberian position that religion provides cultural resources in the form of ultimate meanings that protect the elderly from helplessness and hopelessness. These are the theoretical arguments for statistical tests of the main effect of religious involvement in health (the global hypothesis), and for the indirect effects of religious involvement in health through the three explanatory hypotheses: the behavioral, cohesiveness, and coherence hypotheses.

Chapter II argues that, in addition to these main and indirect effects, religion may also have an interactive effect in modifying the relationship between objective health conditions and the individual's subjective perceptions of them. This is the argument for the theodicy function of religion, its ability to provide meaning for experiences of suffering. The suffering in this case is that caused by the chronic illness and disability of this elderly population, and the argument could be summarized by saying that religion modifies the elderly's subjective perceptions of physical illness/disability. Chapter II, then, introduces the fourth explanatory hypothesis of the study, the theodicy hypothesis. The difference between Chapters I and II turns on the key distinction between the public and private forms of religious involvement, a distinction which will be shown to be of crucial importance in studying the elderly.

Chapter III describes the study design, the measurements, scales, and analytic techniques, and discusses the methodological limitations on the interpretability of the results.

In Chapter IV, initial age, sex, and ethnic-religious differences in religious participation are reported. The findings for the sample are weighted according to census data, and thus represent religious participation patterns among the elderly in New Haven as a whole. There is an analysis of the relationship of the various forms of religious involvement with the indicators that will be used to test the three major hypotheses: the measures of health behaviors, cohesion, and coherence. Short of any relationship with health, the various forms of religious participation may have some interesting associations with particular health habits, certain features of the elderly's social networks, or their senses of coherence, and an understanding of these relationships is a necessary foundation for the later analyses.

Chapters V through VIII report the analyses of the relationships of religious involvement and (respectively) chronic conditions, functional ability, depression, and the subjective assessment of health. The plausibility of the alternative hypotheses are evaluated on the basis of this cross-sectional analysis. It is the comparison of the associations of the various types of religious participation with particular aspects of health and physical functioning that will yield the most important findings.

Chapter IX summarizes the findings within the broader perspective of classical sociological theories of religion, and assesses their usefulness as guides for generating hypotheses for future research. The ultimate goal, toward which this study is only a first step, is to outline a foundation in classical sociological theory for contemporary social epidemiology, one which may provide a framework for advancing our understanding of the health consequences of cultural patterns.

Cohesiveness
and
Coherence

I
On Religion and Health

The Classical Roots of Cohesiveness and Coherence

> . . . while religion, the family and the nation are preservatives against . . . suicide, the cause of this does not lie in the special sort of sentiments encouraged by each. Rather, they all owe this virtue to the general fact that they are societies and they possess it only in so far as they are well integrated societies; that is, without excess in one direction or the other. Quite a different group may, then, have the same effect, if it has the same *cohesion*. Besides the society of faith, of family and of politics, there is one other of which no mention has yet been made; that of all workers of the same sort, in association, all who cooperate in the same function, that is, the occupational group or corporation [my emphasis].
>
> Durkheim (1897, p. 378)

> Even the gods to whom one turns for protection are . . . regarded as either subject to some social and moral order or as the creators of such an order, which they made the specific content of their divine will. In the first case, a superordinate and impersonal power makes its appearance behind the gods, controlling them from within and measuring the value of their deeds. Of course this supra-divine power may take many different forms. It appears first as '*fate*.' Among the Greeks fate (*moira*) is an irrational and, above all, ethically neutral predestination of the fundamental aspects of every man's destiny. The predetermination is elastic within certain limits, but flagrant interferences with predestined fate by wicked maneuvers may imperil even the greatest of the gods . . . This provides one explanation for the failure of so many prayers.

. . . revelation involves . . . a unified view of the world
derived from a consciously integrated and meaningful
attitude toward life. . . .both the life of man and the world,
both social and cosmic events, have a certain systematic
and *coherent meaning*. To this meaning the conduct of
mankind must be oriented if it is to bring salvation, for
only in relation to this meaning does life obtain a unified
and significant pattern. Now the structure of this meaning
may take varied forms, and it may weld together into a
unity motives that are logically quite heterogeneous. The
whole conception is dominated, not by logical consistency,
but by practical valuations. Yet it always denotes,
regardless of any variations in scope and measure of
success, an effort to systematize all the manifestations of
life; that is, to organize practical behavior into a direction
of life, regardless of the form it may assume in any
individual case. Moreover, it always contains the important
religious conception of the world as a cosmos which is
challenged to produce somehow a "meaningful," ordered
totality . . . [my emphasis].

Weber (1922, pp. 36-7, 58-9)

The sociology of religion has not outgrown the depth and
spread of its classical roots. These two selections from Emile
Durkheim's *Suicide* and Max Weber's *The Sociology of Religion* place
the concepts of cohesiveness and coherence squarely in their proper
historical context. They represent the two strands of sociological
thinking about religion that have been present from the inception of the
discipline. Their use in the contemporary social-epidemiological
context, then, carries with it all the richness of insight these traditions
have to offer, and the obligation of acknowledging the debt. Durkheim
and Weber opened up the two main roads along which social scientific
thinking about religion has continued to travel, which Greeley (1982)
has (perhaps too neatly) labelled the "belonging" and "meaning"
functions of religion. To Durkheim it was the holding-power, the
cohesive force, of the religious group that was of primary importance,
not any particular set of beliefs or symbols. What fascinated Weber
were the ways in which characteristic psychological conditions,
produced by the coherent view of the world given by religious belief,
could have historical-social consequences for human activities and
institutions.[1]

For Durkheim, religion was defined as a system of symbols by which individuals in society became conscious of their collective existence. Religion arose from beliefs regarding the sacred and the profane, beliefs Durkheim saw as universal. He characterized religion as an anonymous and diffuse force compelling human beings to believe and worship. What they worship, according to Durkheim, is precisely their collective existence, society itself. His sociology was a study of social facts, among which religion was included. A social fact is a thing, a thing whose most important characteristic is the constraint it exercises on individuals. Durkheim's cohesiveness, then, is the generic form of social force tying the individual to the group.

This idea of religion as an external force compelling human behavior runs in a fundamental opposition to the attempt Weber made to understand life as it is lived. His effort to understand human social action emphasizes above all the subjective meaning of actions. It was his belief that human activity took place in a social context, that "social action is . . . an individual's behavior . . . in relation to the actual or anticipated potential behavior of other individuals" (Weber, 1978, p. 1376). The values that inform human action are products of social collectivities, and as such, may vary from one group to another. Not only may different values arise in different societies, thus introducing the possibility of conflict, but contradictory values may arise within the same society. Religious practices come under the rubric of value-laden, meaningful social action. Religion, as dogma, belief, ritual, and institution is a highly important informant of any society's, and any individual's, world view.

The Durkheimian and Weberian conceptions of religion contrast strongly with each other. The opaque "givenness" of religion as a cohesive force differs from, but also complements a conception of it as a set of values, transparently constituted by human beings in a social context. Both of these approaches have been and will continue to be the guiding influences in the scientific study of religion, encoding more theoretical insight than has as yet been seen.

With regard to the present study, they provide the theoretical background to the study's hypothesis: *Religious involvement will be positively associated with health.*

Could religious belief or participation in a religious group have any effect on an individual's health? The first to ask this question was Durkheim, whose observation that Catholics committed suicide much less often than Protestants led him to the conclusion that the more tightly-knit a social group, the more likely it was to protect its members from taking their own lives. By choosing suicide as the form of mortality to study in association with religion, Durkheim had the methodological advantage of knowing that his measure of religious involvement chronologically preceded his measure of health. Thus although his theory is based on a cross-sectionaı ecologic analysis of suicide rates in various European countries, common sense assures us that the social condition of religious involvement preceded the act of suicide. But even here (and leaving aside the weaknesses of ecologic data) the issue of causality must be called into question: what if some third factor predisposed individuals both to suicide and to Protestantism? Membership in Protestant churches is frequently a result of conversion experiences, so this is not too far-fetched a possibility. The problems of determining causality multiply as the measure of health is expanded to all forms of mortality, and then to morbidity. And they become even greater as the measure of religious involvement expands from the more permanent nominal affiliation to the changeable activities of religious involvement.

One need ask if an individual's health is also likely to have a bearing on his or her religious activities. Ill health could just as easily (and more self-evidently) cause infrequent religious observance as the other way around. If ill health has limited the population of religious participators before the study begins, a selection effect is operating, and to the extent that a selection effect occurs, it reverses the causal direction. Several methodological ways of reducing causal ambiguity are built into this study, including measuring not only public participation in religious activities but private religious feelings as well, and building controls for physical health status into the measures of disability, depression, and subjective assessment of health. These methods will be covered in detail in Chapter III.

Ultimately, however, methodological safeguards on the inference of causality can never be perfect. The preferred basis for understanding causality must be an empirically testable theoretical conception of the processes by which the causality in question could be accomplished. One must not only ask, is religion associated with health, but why might that be?

The remainder of Chapter I considers three theoretical explanations or mediating processes by which religious involvement could conceivably have an effect on human health: the *behavioral hypothesis*, the *cohesiveness hypothesis*, and the *coherence hypothesis*. The related bodies of literature in epidemiology, sociology, and social psychology are reviewed and discussed, and the groundwork is laid for operationalizing the measures used to test these hypotheses. Chapter I concludes by critically reviewing the rather small number of studies which have looked at religious involvement as a factor in morbidity and mortality studies, summarizing what is known about the relationship and placing the question of religious involvement and health within the larger context of psychosocial factors in health.

The Behavioral Hypothesis

The most straightforward reason that religious involvement might appear to benefit health is the possibility that people in religious groups may behave differently than others with respect to known health risk factors. For religious reasons, certain behaviors may be engaged in or refrained from which then subsequently have health effects. Berkman and Syme (1979) considered this possibility in their study of social networks and mortality. While they do not detail the specific relationship of religious group membership to health practices, they did find social networks in general to be positively associated with a cumulative index of seven health practices, a relationship which diminished, but did not eliminate the original relationship between social networks and mortality. Langlie (1977) looked at types of social networks and their relationship to direct and indirect preventive health behaviors, and found that Protestants, and people whose networks were made up largely of non-kin were more likely to engage in indirect preventive health behavior (using seat belts, getting check-ups) than were Catholics and the more family-centered.

There are numerous specific health practices known to be prescribed or proscribed by certain religious groups. The Baptists of Evans County, Georgia (Graham et al., 1978), Mormons in Utah, (Gardner and Lyon 1982a, 1982b), and Seventh-Day Adventists are known to be nonsmokers, and the health effects of their practice have been noted. Many Protestant denominations, particularly fundamentalists, proscribe drinking (Gardner and Lyon 1982a, 1982b; Wynder, Lemon and Bross, 1959; Hadaway, Elifson, Petersen, 1984); Seventh-Day Adventists are also often vegetarian (Wynder, Lemon and Bross, 1959), as are some Roman Catholic Orders (Groen et al., 1962).

Comstock and Partridge note the lower rates of sexually-transmitted diseases among women attending church frequently, attributing it to ". . . the inverse correlation of church attendance and number of extra-marital coital contacts" (1972, p. 668). Gardner and Lyon (1982), however, could find no differences in cervical cancer in Mormon women with higher church activity levels. As religious practices, these are all *pro*scribed activities. One *pre*scribed religious activity, however, that has been thought to convey beneficial health effects is the enforced rest on the seventh day (Brigham, 1835, p. 315), although this has not to my knowledge been considered by epidemiologists.

As an explanation of the relationship between religion and health, this behavioral mechanism could be expected to have its strongest effect in religiously-homogeneous study populations, where all religiously-related health practice norms would be the same. In such a community, religious involvement could be said to stand for adherence to religious/health practices (Gardner and Lyon, 1982a). In a study of a religiously pluralistic urban community, however, one would expect few if any doctrinally-based sample-wide relationships of religious involvement to specific health practices.

Nevertheless, in this study, four health practices (smoking, alcohol consumption, obesity, and exercise) will be tested for their relationship with religious involvement, and as potential mediators of the relationship between religious involvement and health.

The *behavioral hypothesis* states that the relationship between religious involvement and health is explained by the performance of religiously pre- or proscribed health behaviors which decrease known health risk factors.

The Cohesiveness Hypothesis

The passage from *Suicide* at the beginning of the chapter contains all the elements of the argument for the cohesiveness hypothesis. Durkheim's thesis is that religion has a preservative effect against the egoistic type of suicide, not because of any particular sentiments it arouses, but because an individual's membership in the body of believers is an attachment to an integrated social group. "religion, the family and the nation . . . all owe this virtue [their apparent effect in preventing suicide] to the general fact that they are societies." With regard to the health of the elderly, then, under this hypothesis religious group involvement should be salutary *because* it is, and only in so far as it is social group involvement. Thus it is the public, sociable, service-attending aspects of religious group involvement that should be associated with health, not the private, solitary aspects. This is the part of Durkheim's argument that is remembered by the researchers who find "social support" a sufficient description of the functions of social networks.

But there was another type of suicide that was just as important to Durkheim's theory, and that was anomic suicide, caused by insufficient social regulation. By regulation is meant external social constraint on individual desires. These desires, Durkheim believed, would otherwise be insatiable. Social groups not only surround, comfort, and support, they also demand, control and compel. Most of the current social support literature remains very naive on this point, in not recognizing that the control and regulation of the social group may be just as important for individual well-being as the integration it gives. And it is precisely its ethical demands which are a religion's distinguishing features. Unlike a family, where moral requirements are largely individually-controlled, subject to change and development, the moral requirements, that is the constraints, of religious group membership are historical, traditional, canonized. In some Protestant churches, the fulfillment of ethical demands may be the very condition of membership. There is thus more to religious group membership than simply the pleasantness of sociability.

The cohesiveness hypothesis postulates religious group involvement as an environmental resource in health in much the same way as the current social network-social support literature does, only broadening the conceptualization of its functioning to include regulation as well as integration. The key question is whether religious participation is distinguishable from general social participation. If it is not distinguishable then one would expect church attendance and social involvement in general to be associated with each other and with health.

It is by now a commonplace that social factors have some effect in health. The social network-social support literature is very disparate and growing rapidly. And although current interest in these topics is high, the ideas they are based on are not new. The research on social networks and social support in health is anchored to major bodies of empirical sociological research, in addition to the discipline's major classical theory tradition. The following review of the literature, then, must be highly selected. The best way to distinguish the following studies is with a categorization based on the level of analysis of the relationship between the individual and the environment, calling the levels macro, mezzo, and micro.[2]

The macro level of population analysis could be said to have started in this country with Faris and Dunham's (1939) study of mental disorder in Chicago. They used, as did Durkheim in *Suicide*, an ecologic analysis, the correlation of rates within geographically-divided areas. They found the highest overall insanity rates, rates of schizophrenia and alcoholic psychosis to be most heavily concentrated in the disorganized, deteriorated center of the city, especially where many people lived in rooming-houses. Though regarded as a classic, there are serious biases in the study's ecologic analysis and use of treatment rates. This study is probably most important because it gave rise to the social causation-social selection controversy (Wheaton, 1978). But it also for the first time associated mental disorder with isolation, the absence of social networks and supports, and advanced a plausible, if untested, explanation for that association--that "the seclusive person is freed from the social control which enforces normality in other people (Faris and Dunham, 1967 [1939], p. 174). The Berkman and Syme (1979) and House, Robbins, and Metzner (1982) studies discussed earlier are the most recent and methodologically sophisticated of this type. Studies carried out at this level measure the absence or presence of an individual's social networks, differentiated at most by nominal type, and their relationship to the individual's health. But they do not probe the mechanisms of social support, nor specific instances in which it did or did not occur. In both studies, various types of formal and informal social relations were included, and their apparent functional interchangeability was noted by Berkman and Syme (1979), ". . . it was only in the absence of either of these source of contacts that there was a significant increase in the risk of death during the follow-up period" (p. 201). House, Robbins, and Metzner's (1982) study had more mixed results, finding more kinds of social relationships significantly associated with mortality for men than for women. Their finding of no association at all between mortality and *satisfaction* in relationships, as does Faris and Dunham's "enforcement of normality," confirms the two-edged Durkheimian view that there is more to social life than social rewards.

If research at the macro level can be said to determine whether or not the social environment plays any role at all in health, the mezzo level is most concerned with specifying its structure, function, and when it comes into play: the who, how, and when questions. Kaplan, Cassel, and Gore (1977) call the structural and functional aspects the morphological and interactional properties. With regard to the former, health researchers have had the benefit of the work of a generation of social network researchers in anthropology, beginning with Elizabeth Bott (1957) and developing through Mitchell (1969), Barnes (1972), Boissevain and Mitchell (1973), all of whom were concerned with problems other than health. This research has generated a sophisticated, quantitatively precise way of carving up the social body, by looking at the social network's density, range, size, homogeneity, multiplexity. Given this high level of conceptual development, it is surprising that so few health researchers have focused their efforts here. Many more have been drawn to the interactional-functional end of the problem. Focusing on the health correlates of the purely structural aspects of networks, however, could be very interesting, both as a general problem and specifically with regard to religion. Laumann's (1973) study of the structures of the social networks of 1013 white Detroit men found religious preference to be associated with distinctly different network structures. Catholics were more likely to have networks of friends who were ethnically and religiously like themselves than Protestants were. This sameness, or "ethnoreligious homogeneity" is also associated with longer duration of friendship, and with interlocking (or closed-circle), rather than radial (or open-circle) friendship networks. Laumann concludes ". . . religious differences appear in general to have a much stronger impact on the compositional homogeneity of a man's friendship network than his socioeconomic status characteristics" (p. 108). If religious group involvement is found to be related to health, these social network characteristics may be as well. The conceptualizations of positive-negative ties (Wellman, 1981) and strong-weak ties (Granovetter, 1973) may also prove very useful in analyzing religion's place in the social network.

It is the functioning of this structure that has been addressed by the social support literature, which has often taken the how and the when questions simultaneously. Heavily influenced by the life events tradition in mental health research, (Holmes and Rahe, 1967; Dohrenwend and Dohrenwend, 1974), the first social support investigations tended to focus on the provision of aid in stressful life event situations (Nuckolls, Cassel, and Kaplan, 1972; Myers, Lindenthal, and Pepper, 1975; Gore, 1978). These early findings led many to make assumptions which should instead have been open questions. The overriding question has been, does social support buffer the effects of life event stress on health? In other words, more attention has been directed at the context of support than at its content. (Detailed reviews of these studies can be found in Cobb, 1976; Dean and Lin, 1977; Mueller, 1980).

The major problems with studying social support as a buffer against life stress have recently been reviewed by Thoits (1982). She argues that most studies have lacked a precise conceptual definition of social support, implying that they also lack a theoretical perspective on the problem. This has permitted *post hoc* analyses and a proliferation of off-the-cuff operationalizations, all contributing to the conceptual anarchy. The multidimensionality of the concept further complicates the issue. Most importantly, she argues that the difficulties of studying life events in conjunction with social support have been gravely underestimated because the two are conceptually, if not methodologically, confounded. In other words, in some way, social support networks and the subjects of life events are exactly the same thing. Many of the most important life events are gains or losses of supportive relationships, entrances or exits from the social field, which change simultaneously the situation and the resources to deal with the situation. Even measuring social support at one point in time and life events at a later time cannot eliminate the effects of life events on social support because social support at any time is the product of previous life events. She concludes that social support may have a main causal effect of its own, in addition to, or instead of interacting with life event stress. That is, rather than coming into play only in the presence of one or more life crises, social supports may exert a constant influence of their own.

Treating social support as an etiological factor in itself will compel better operationalization and conceptualization. Unfortunately, most extant studies have reduced social support, intentionally but nevertheless naively, to emotional support (Dean and Lin, 1977; Gore, 1978; Blazer, 1982; LaRocco, House, and French, 1980). At this stage of research, the multidimensionality of the concept requires that all kinds of aid be included, instrumental, financial, informational, task assistance, as well as social and emotional aid, if the full range   of expression of support is to be accounted for. Kaplan, Cassel, and Gore, (1977) define social support comprehensively as ". . . gratification of a person's basic social needs" (p. 50). In social network language, the ties are multi-stranded. The implication of these broader measures, and of the main effect argument in general is that social supports are more ubiquitous than sporadic crisis resources, that they either have some independent positive effect of their own, or they are continually modifying the lower levels of non-crisis, daily life stress.

A current tally of studies finding buffering effects or main effects calls the conclusion an open question (Wheaton, 1983). Of 22 recent studies, seven found some evidence for an interaction effect, but 15 found a main effect only (p. 210). Though the evidence would appear to be stronger for the main effect side, it is important to note that four of the seven studies which found an interaction effect did not find the interaction with life event stress at all, but with the everyday, chronic stress condition of work. This suggests that interactions between life stress and social supports are more likely to be found in cases of specific, identified stressful conditions. The view taken in the present study is that both main and interactive effects are plausible and significantly different enough from each other that it is important to know if each or both are present. But the infinite regress of causation between life events and social supports discussed above precludes the possibility of a final answer. Social support must be considered a dynamic force, not a static condition, the subject of change as well as the author of it. A great deal could be learned, however, if main and interaction effects were both tested in various situations of specific stresses, and questions of ultimate causation left aside. Consistently, these studies have had the strongest results (Nuckolls, Cassel, and Kaplan, 1971; Kasl, Gore, and Cobb, 1975; Liem and Liem, 1978; LaRocco, House and French, 1980; Turner, 1981). Such an approach, which will be the one taken here, could be particularly revealing in studies of the elderly, who suffer proportionately more of the most highly stressful life events and conditions, particularly bereavement and illness.

A third important level of analysis, the micro level, is composed of studies that concern the individual and just his or her most important primary relationships. These studies are often more qualitative than quantitative, more focused on the process of interaction than its structure or outcome. Beginning with Bowlby's (1969) germinal work on the nature and development of human attachment, these researchers have often used the disturbed attachments of psychiatric patients as a counterpoint for understanding normal attachment. For example, Pattison et al. (1975) found the primary groups of their neurotic subjects to be smaller, less interconnected, and more often rated negatively than those of normal subjects. Very similar results were obtained by Henderson et al. (1978) in another study, where it was also found that patients considered their primary attachments to be giving them insufficient support. Perhaps most important, however, is the presence of a single close relationship, that of an intimate confidant. Lowenthal and Haven (1968) found the presence or absence of an intimate relationship to be the single most important factor associated with psychiatric impairment and morale in a sample of elderly subjects. A large number of less intimate social relationships was not an effective substitute. Brown and Harris (1978) found the presence of a confidant to be one of the most important factors protecting women suffering severe life events from becoming depressed. Studies at this level establish the foundations of social support, the fund of sociability (Weiss, 1969).

Given these known associations of social networks and social supports with health, the cohesiveness hypothesis postulates that it is because religious group involvement is simply another form of social group involvement that it is associated with health. Although I have consistently identified this argument as Durkheimian, Durkheim was actually more subtle in his understanding of religion. In *Suicide*, he does argue that it is not religion which produces the cohesive society, but rather the cohesion itself which seems religious, but he also constantly uses differences in the suicide rates of Protestants, Catholics, and Jews to illustrate differences in anomic and egoistic suicide. The three vary in the strength of their cohesiveness:

> The more numerous and strong these collective states of mind are, the stronger the integration of the religious community, and also the greater its preservative value. The details of dogmas and rites are secondary. The essential thing is that they be capable of supporting a sufficiently intense collective life. And because the Protestant church has less consistency than the others it has less moderating effect upon suicide (1951, p. 170).

Is religious participation functionally interchangeable with social participation with respect to health? In the Berkman and Syme (1979) study it was, to a certain extent. Other studies have found significant associations of health with religious, but not other voluntary group memberships (House, Robbins, and Metzner, 1982; Cutler, 1976). If it is not functionally interchangeable, what are the social-structural or social-interactional qualities that differentiate religious group participation from other groups, and also that differentiate one religious group from another? Several characteristics of the religious group suggest that there may be some differences: the uniqueness of the social network structure of the religious group, its institutional legitimacy, and the ritualistic nature of the social interaction within it.

A network characteristic that speaks for the uniqueness of the religious group is most directly a consequence of its size. Most individuals' relationships to a religious group will be made up of a mixture of strong and weak ties. Strong ties are usually presumed to be more emotionally supportive, intense, and of longer duration. Weak ties have been less appreciated, but they have been shown to have their own important functions in the transmission of information and the integration of the individual into the larger society (Granovetter, 1973). Moreover, most religious group's members span the entire age range, which is not true of many modern social institutions. Religious group involvement may derive its protectiveness from this multifunctionality of ties; membership in a religious group, like membership in a large extended family, may provide one with intimate emotional ties, distant instrumental ones, and the potential for the provision of many of the dimensions of social support.

The relative proportions of strong and weak ties may well vary by religious group. Laumann's (1973) research noted above found great differences in the homogeneity of the friendship networks of Catholics and Protestants. Glock and Stark (1965) took an even closer look by comparing Protestant denominations. They found not a single Congregationalist in their sample to have all four or five of his or her best friends belonging to the same church, while significant proportions of the more conservative Baptist and Methodist church members did. Moreover, they found a significant positive association between friendship involvement and the intensity of an individual's religious experience, a truly Durkheimian finding.

The second characteristic is the ability of the institution to influence human behavior in the direction of supporting and caring for others. Durkheim puts it, not ethically, but sociologically,

> . . . the believer feels that he is obliged to accept certain forms of behavior imposed on him by the nature of the sacred principle with which he feels he is in communication. But society also maintains in us the sensation of a perpetual dependence, because it has a nature peculiar to itself, different from our individual nature, and pursues ends which are likewise peculiar to itself; but since it can attain them only through us, it imperiously demands our cooperation. It requires that we forget our personal interests and become its servants; it subjects us to all kinds of inconveniences, hardships, and sacrifices without which social life should be impossible. So it is that at every moment we are obliged to submit to rules of conduct and ideas which we have neither made nor willed and which are sometimes even opposed to our most fundamental inclinations and instincts (Aron, 1967, p. 51).

The passage underlines the compelling externality of the religious institution, its social power in overriding individual interests. The power, of course, rests on the strength of individual commitment to the group, a commitment which may be based on cognitive, emotional, or moral claims (Kanter, 1968). It is true that the consequences of religion for the individual in modern society may be more of the "reward" than the "responsibility" variety (Glock and Stark, 1965), but there are nevertheless significant moral requirements for religious group membership.

The third characteristic of the religious group is its ritual. Although American Protestantism may have reduced the role of ritual in the religious service to a minimum, even here the behavior of religious worship is highly ritualized behavior. Religious ritual is a social situation structured to produce religious experience (Glock and Stark, 1965). It provides a frame for that experience, with a beginning, a middle, and an end (Douglas, 1966; Van Gennep, 1960 [1908]). Whatever the content of the ritual, there is always some physical, bodily aspect. One important group of rituals, rites of passage, often have disfiguration or scarification as an element. Even the more benign practices, for instance baptism or communion, involve physical experiences of several of the senses. Both ritual and meditation have been shown to coordinate the brain and the body (d'Aquili, Laughlin, and McManus, 1979) by focusing the attention on a rhythmic movement or chant. Healing rituals are especially focused on the body, an experience which unifies momentarily the symbolic, the social, and the physical, and gives religious meaning to the experience of illness (McGuire, 1982). The anthropological view has been that rituals function for the benefit of the social group (Malinowski, 1948; Radcliffe-Brown, 1952 [1939]; Turner, 1967). They enact human, social control over the material world. In general, ritual has integrative functions for the social group as a whole: it reduces interpersonal conflict, reminds the group of its traditions, reinforces its values, and strengthens the bonds within it.

The cohesiveness hypothesis, then, draws on the Durkheimian sociological tradition to argue that it is the social bonds tying the individual to the social group that are responsible for the association of religious involvement and health. The tightness with which they knit may vary from one religious group to another, but it is the range and closeness of ties and social support they make available to the individual that is important. Thus it is the public, religious-service-attending aspect of religious involvement that should be most strongly associated with health.

The *cohesiveness hypothesis* states that the relationship between religious involvement and health is explained by the social networks and social support of the religious group.

The Coherence Hypothesis

The coherence hypothesis makes the argument for a positive association between religion and health at the cognitive level, a level of explanation that is finding increased emphasis in all the social sciences (Proudfoot and Shaver, 1975). Rooted in the Weberian imperative to understand human action at the level of its meaning, this approach has informed the best contemporary work in the sociology of religion (Douglas, 1966; Berger, 1967; Bellah, 1970; Geertz, 1973). Not one of these writers, however, has written on health. And from the epidemiological side, studies with a cognitive emphasis have usually not considered religion (Hinkle and Wolff, 1958; Cassel and Tyroler, 1961; Leighton et al., 1963; Tyroler and Cassel, 1964). What has been lacking is an adequate social psychology capable of analyzing processes in both religion and health. Thus what follows is a exploratory attempt to outline a cognitive social psychology of religion that has implications for health. The coherence hypothesis, in a word, is that religion as a system of symbols provides cultural resources in the form of a consistent body of knowledge and set of meanings that allows individuals to make sense of and cope with their experience. Religion provides cultural resources to individuals by making available socially shared, spiritually based means of interpretation for *all* the events of life, reducing uncertainty in ordinary daily life and at moments of crisis alike. Coherence is the sense that life, at its high points and lows, is meaningful and can be understood, if not controlled. It is thus individual and private by comparison with the social interaction of the cohesiveness hypothesis, but it is not an idiosyncratic personal resource in the sense of a character trait. It is a cultural resource in that the meanings of its symbols are historical, traditional, and shared.

The origins of the cognitive approach in epidemiology are found in the work of John Cassel, a South African physician who studied the health effects of culture change in North Carolina. In one study (Cassel and Tyroler, 1961) it was found that the industrialization of a previously rural agricultural community had the most severe health consequences (in the form of days absent from work and score on the Cornell Medical Index) for the "first generation" factory workers, those whose parents were farmers. At the same time, second generation workers, who had grown up in the homes of factory workers and for whom the routines of factory workers' lives were familiar, had significantly better health status. Their second study looked at the effect of rapid urban growth in all the counties of North Carolina and compared it by means of the coronary heart disease mortality in those counties (Tyroler and Cassel, 1964). They found the highest CHD mortality rates among the rural residents of the most rapidly urbanizing counties, the group which presumably was experiencing the most culture change. Their interpretation of the findings, in general, was that changes in social systems are stressful to individuals when their cultural norms are no longer appropriate, when their "designs for living" are inadequate (Cassel, Patrick, and Jenkins, 1960). In their words, the key question is "How effectively has the past experience of this group equipped it to cope with its present life situation?" (p. 949)

Aaron Antonovsky (1979) uses the concept of a sense of coherence to further a highly Cassel-influenced interpretation[3] of his and others' research on stress and coping in health. His use of the concept is in some ways similar to the way it is used here. He defines the sense of coherence as ". . . a global orientation that expresses the extent to which one has a pervasive, enduring though dynamic feeling of confidence that one's internal and external environments are predictable and that there is a high probability that things will work out as well as can reasonably be expected" (p. 10). The two elements that comprise the sense of coherence he calls predictability and lawfulness. As in Cassel's work, religion plays little role. He identifies three sources of the sense of coherence: the psychological (stemming from early childhood experiences); social structural (mainly from the complexity of work conditions); and cultural-historical (in that cultures produce personality types). However, he finds individual differences in the extent of senses of coherence so great as to tip the balance in favor of the psychological explanation based on child-rearing patterns (p. 191). The concept of coherence I am trying to develop here differs from Antonovsky's in its constituent elements and hence its definition to a certain extent, but mostly it differs in its origins. The concept of coherence as I am using it refers to the conscious activities of adults in interpreting the significance of their life situations, not to a predisposing psychological characteristic that is set in place in early childhood. The question of whether early socialization or adult religious beliefs are more powerful in shaping one's sense of coherence is ultimately an empirical question, one which certainly cannot be addressed with the present data. Moreover, to my knowledge, Antonovsky has not operationalized his concept, making the present attempt to do so purely exploratory. In any event, the term coherence as Weber used it conveys exactly the sense I intend: that of ". . . a unified view of the world derived from a consciously integrated and meaningful attitude toward life."

While the cognitive approach has been relatively rare in epidemiological studies of physical illness, its use in psychology has been very influential, producing an important new theory of the origins of depression. As it has developed, the theory of learned helplessness and its reformulation have proved useful both to clinicians and to epidemiologists studying social factors in mental health, two groups whose perspectives are usually very far apart. Having only that to recommend the theory is a great deal, but it has the added advantage of being empirically testable.

Seligman's (1975) theory of learned helplessness was a direct descendent of the cognitive approach to depression of Beck (1967), who identified a cognitive "primary triad" in depression of negative views of the self, the world, and the future. As Beck described him, the depressed individual sees himself as defective or deficient, and rejects himself; he sees others as having derogatory ideas about him; and he sees only hardship and suffering in the future. This emphasis on the patient's perception was a new way to look at depression. Seligman, a student of Beck, theorizing on the basis of laboratory experiments with animals, formulated the learned helplessness hypothesis: that learning that outcomes are uncontrollable produces three kinds of deficits: motivational, cognitive, and emotional (Seligman, 1975).

Since 1975 Seligman and his colleagues have revised, or reformulated the theory with the analytic advantage of attribution theory. The reformulation of the learned helplessness hypothesis extends the analysis primarily at the cognitive level (Abramson, Seligman, and Teasdale, 1978). Briefly stated, the reformulated theory contends that helplessness results when the individual comes to believe that there is nothing he can do to prevent something bad from happening, or to cause something desired to occur. Individuals in such situations will ask themselves why they are helpless, and the causes to which they attribute their difficulties will determine the generality and chronicity of their helplessness, how widely it will spread through other aspects of their life, and how long the feelings of helplessness last. Individuals who interpret their failures as being the result of stable, global, and internal factors are at much higher risk of depression than individuals who attribute failures to external, specific, and unstable factors.

The development of attribution theory has proceeded by refining the categories with which individuals interpret their experiences, their behavior, and the behavior of others. Beginning with Heider's "naive psychology" (1958), Festinger's cognitive dissonance (Festinger, Riecken, Schachter, 1956), Rotter's (1966) work on internal versus external control of reinforcement, Kelley's mental analyses of variance (1967), and Weiner's causal determinants of ability, effort, task difficulty, and luck (1972), many streams have flowed into this pool. It is not necessary to develop any of these individual theories, only to note the important conclusion that all took steps toward: that causal determinations made in certain situations generalize to other situations. This issue of generalization has more often been assumed than proved (Wortman and Brehm, 1975) and yet it goes directly to the very meaning of the condition of helplessness. Only if attributions of helplessness in one situation have some tendency to spread to other situations does the helplessness theory have relevance to any larger condition of depression. The idea of generalization also suggests that there are some predictable patterns by which attributions will be distributed, and this is the way in which attribution theory becomes relevant to religion and to a sense of coherence.

One of the chief limitations of attribution theory for the study of religion has arisen from its development in laboratory experiments with subjects engaged in success/failure trials (Lazarus and Launier, 1978; Coyne, Aldwin, and Lazarus, 1981). The laboratory situations the subjects encountered contained unique, novel, and short-lived stresses. Presumably the investigators chose loud noises and electric shocks because they considered them uniformly stressful, but that deprived subjects of the ability to cope with the event at the level of its meaning by interpreting the situation in familiar terms. Moreover, the attributions studied were made in the context of achievement-oriented situations in which the perceived causes of the success or failure could be exhaustively and mutually exclusively described by the categories of ability, effort, task difficulty, and luck (Weiner, 1972). Built into the theory is the presumption that the life-situations to which these attributions generalize contain the possibility of completely successful resolution. One author decries responses in which "more time may be expended in prayer, gambling, or search for succor than at instrumental acts that could help to create the desired ends (Lefcourt, 1980, p. 247). I believe it has been the social psychologists' need to control the situation that has caused them to limit their attention to the narrow concept of failure and ignore the wider concept of misfortune. (This limitation is openly acknowledged by Abramson, Seligman, and Teasdale, (1977, p. 55) and Weiner (1972, p. 374)). It has also made necessary the logical gymnastics about a so-called "illusion of control": the perception that an individual succeeded due to his own effort/ability when the outcome was veridically noncontingent (as outcomes in real life often are) (Langer, 1983).

Situational attributions are relevant to the study of religion only as indications of characteristic attributions, and the more unrepresentative the situation in which they are elicited, the less likely they are to indicate their characteristic. In fact, exactly how characteristic an individual's attributions are ought to be a major question. For these reasons, then, the attribution-theory-based concept of fatalism (Wheaton, 1983; Lefcourt, cited in Wortman and Brehm, 1975) places the characteristic attributions at a more suitably generalizable level. Drawing on Kohn's (1972) concept of an "orientational system," Wheaton has defined fatalism as an "organizing construct" (1983, p. 214) that links and generalizes the concepts of learned helplessness, external locus of control and powerlessness. An individual whose characteristic attributions are fatalistic sees more efficacy in the environment than in himself. He does not, however, (and this is a very important point) necessarily view the environment as hostile. Impenetrability does not imply perniciousness. Wheaton (1980) has invoked the concept of fatalism to explain the known effect of low socioeconomic status on psychological disorder. In a more recent study (Wheaton, 1983), fatalism and inflexibility, considered as indicators of coping effort and ability, jointly reduce the effects of stress, both chronic and acute, on depression. Fatalism, then, is a characteristic attribution that has been shown to be associated with psychological distress. It is here considered one of two characteristic attributions which indicate the presence or absence of a sense of coherence. Fatalism, or rather its inverse form, instrumentalism, is the first of two characteristic attributions that I would like to propose as components of the sense of coherence; the other is the attribution of meaning.

Kohn's (1972) original concept of an orientational system, defined as ". . . conceptions of the external world and of self that serve to define men's stance toward reality" (p. 300), is considerably broader in scope than the single fatalism construct. The orientational system is better viewed as a coordinated set of characteristic attributions which may include fatalism and inflexibility, but also includes another element that has not been given subsequent attention. In Kohn's words,

> the lower a man's social-class position, the more likely is his orientational system to be marked by a rigidly conservative view of man and his social institutions, fearfulness and distrust, and a fatalistic belief that one is at the mercy of forces and people beyond one's control, often, *beyond one's understanding*" (p. 300, my emphasis).

He then quotes Rainwater's (1968) review of studies which comes to a similar conclusion:

> All investigators who have studied lower-class groups seem to come up with compatible findings to the general effect that the lower-class world view involves conceptions of the world as *a hostile and relatively chaotic place* in which you have to be always on guard, a place in which one must be careful about trusting others, in which the reward for effort expended is always problematic, in which good intentions net very little" (p. 241, my emphasis).

Wheaton (1980, p. 104) has argued that fatalistic attributions do not include a sense of meaninglessness, or the lack of understanding and perceptions of chaos Kohn and Rainwater refer to. In fact, there is no logically necessary relation between the two. A belief in the salience of environmental causation and corresponding sense of individual *help*lessness need not imply *hope*lessness if the environment is perceived as benign or at least predictable. Meaninglessness is a characteristic attribution that could be said to be concerned more with the very existence of causality than with its location. Attributing causality to an event implies some understanding of it, some placement of it within a pattern, even if it is a pattern of good or bad luck. Correspondingly, attribution of causality is a denial that events are random, chaotic, and without order. Thus, in a sense the dimension of meaninglessness gets at the fundamental question of just how characteristic and generalizable an individual's attributions are. While it is possible to be helpless without being hopeless, it is not possible to be hopeless without also being helpless (Garber, Miller, and Abramson, 1980).

The early critiques of the helplessness concept focused on the concept's inadequacy, (stemming from its use in potentially controllable experimental situations) in explaining the coping behavior of individuals in truly uncontrollable situations. Wortman and Brehm (1975) note that there are many life situations in which people have no option of exercising control, and that repeated attempts to gain control when one is veridically helpless could be very frustrating and maladaptive. Indeed this is the first major issue addressed the Abramson, Seligman, and Teasdale (1978) reformulation of the learned helplessness theory, the distinction between universal and personal helplessness. The attribution of meaning or meaninglessness in situations with truly uncontrollable outcomes, that is, outcomes about which one would be realistically fatalistic, is thus especially important.

What does it mean to give meaning to experience? What follows is an exploratory attempt to decompose the activity of meaning-giving, with and without reference to religion. As a new construct it requires a formal definition. *Attributing meaning to a situation is the activity of defining the subject in terms of and organizing it according to a scheme of values, beliefs, and symbols that contains the potential for generating causal and moral judgments, with the effect that the individual sees his experience as shared and relativizes his experience by de-individualizing it.*

Attributing meaning to a situation is the activity of . . .

The key word in the phrase is "activity." As long ago as 1932, in a series of experiments on the recall of stories and pictures, Bartlett observed in his subjects an "effort after meaning," ". . . a constant effort to get the maximum possible of meaning into the material present" (Bartlett, 1932, p. 84). The importance of "activeness," initiative, in the process has been more recently observed by Chanowitz and Langer (1980) with their distinction between mindlessness and mindfulness. Their argument is that "mindful" control of material is more psychologically beneficial than "mindless" control, even if the behavior and outcome are identical. It is the active creation of distinctions that makes the experience enlivening. The giving of meaning to a situation is similarly conceived as an active, conscious process, though whether or not it confers psychological benefit as does the experience of control (Langer, 1983) remains to be seen.

. . . defining the subject in terms of and organizing it according to a scheme . . .

Bartlett's (1932) "effort after meaning" entailed "connecting a given pattern with some setting or schema" (p. 20) other than itself, for the purpose of "rendering material acceptable, understandable, comfortable, straightforward; to rob it of all puzzling elements" (p. 89). More recently Douglas (1966) has put it this way:

> In a chaos of shifting impressions, each of us constructs a stable world in which objects have recognizable shapes, are located in depth, and have permanence. In perceiving we are building, taking some cues and rejecting others. The most acceptable cues are those which fit most easily into the pattern that is being built up. Ambiguous ones tend to be treated as if they harmonized with the rest of the pattern. Discordant ones tend to be rejected. If they are accepted the structure of assumptions has to be modified (p. 36).

Chanowitz and Langer (1980) also discuss the structures that emerge from an accumulation of mindful encounters. While religion is an obvious example of a belief scheme, such schemes need not be religious. In a study of what they call "ultimate values," McCready and Greeley (1976) identify four "interpretive responses to life problems," only one of which is necessarily religious: 1) religious optimism, 2) hopefulness, 3) secular optimism, and 4) pessimism. These are "ultimate" schema in that they are only called on when routine interpretive schemes cannot be used. Allport's term for a similar concept is the "master sentiment," among which he finds the religious sentiment the most comprehensive:

> . . . whenever in a mature personality a mature religious sentiment does develop it has a heavy duty to perform, for it is charged with the task of accommodating every atom of experience that is referred to it. Other master sentiments are ordinarily less ambitious in their scope. . . . the mature religious sentiment lays itself open to all facts, to all values, and disvalues and claims to have the clue to their theoretical and practical inclusion in a frame of life (Allport, 1950, p. 54).

This issue of the relative inclusiveness of religious and nonreligious schemes will be taken up again in the second chapter. Here it is enough to say that interpretive frames may or may not be religious in nature.

. . . of values, beliefs, and symbols . . .

Meaning-giving is conceived here as an individual activity, but it is not idiosyncratic. The frameworks are accumulated over the individual's life-history but their structure is delimited by the culture in which they are formed. Culture is used here in the sense of Geertz: "an historically transmitted pattern of meanings embodied in symbols, a system of inherited conceptions expressed in symbolic forms by means of which men communicate, perpetuate, and develop their knowledge about and attitudes toward life" (1973, p. 89). Again, symbols may be but need not be religious; symbols are anything that serves as a vehicle for conception. Symbols are more powerful as conceptions than that which they refer to because they can more easily be held in the mind.

. . . that contains the potential for generating causal . . .

One of the most consistent findings in attribution research has been that people are very reluctant to attribute outcomes to chance (Walster, 1966). Even when the outcome could not possibly have been caused by the individual, there is a bias toward finding some causal agency somewhere. Wortman and Brehm (1975) note that there must be some psychological benefit in making causal attributions in such situations. They note the otherwise puzzling tendency of parents to blame themselves for their children's fatal leukemias (Chodoff, Friedman, and Hamburg, 1964), an evidently adaptive response. The frameworks structure causal attributions in situations of failure and misfortune by identifying sources of threat in the environment and in the self. They nurture, channel, and limit responses. They enable the individual to think of reasons why and why not. They act to reduce areas of uncertainty in which attributions would have to be made to luck or chance, by imputing causal agency to the self or an identifiable feature of the environment.

. . . and moral judgments . . .

The moral content of causal attributions has been recognized from the start. A long series of experiments (beginning with Lerner, 1970, and summarized in Rubin and Peplau, 1975; and Langer, 1983), has shown widespread evidence of the general belief that people get what they deserve, another way of reducing uncertainty. Sometimes called the "just world theory," it has been used most often to explain the behavior of blaming the victim when the victim could not possibly have been at fault. The belief in a just world has been correlated in different studies with religiousness, authoritarianism, and an internal locus of control (Rubin and Peplau, 1975). Kelley (1971), in an interesting attributional analysis of moral evaluation, outlines three moral bases for evaluation: reality, achievement, and reciprocity, suggesting that ideas of what "ought" to be are greatly influenced by what "is."

> *. . . with the effect that the individual*
> *sees his experience as shared . . .*

The frameworks are built up out of elements of the culture, ensuring some similarity of frameworks within groups. Group schemata condition what the individual perceived in the environment and the permissible parameters of possible response. The necessity of social support in maintaining beliefs is most dramatically illustrated when those beliefs are not widely shared (Festinger, Riecken, Schachter, 1964 [1956]). However dangerous it may seem to some psychologists (Kelley, 1971), most people's beliefs, knowledge, and moral judgments are socially constructed (Berger and Luckmann, 1967).

> *. . . and relativizes his experience by de-individualizing it.*

By using the socially available templates for ordering his personal experience, the individual shuffles his personal biography into the history of his society. He comes to view his experiences as moments of human experience, enabling him to transcend any sense of uniqueness and isolation. Giving meaning to a situation transforms it from personal circumstance to typical case. It places it in a context of other situations more and less difficult than itself, and makes available the range of human coping responses that are more and less effective, more and less appropriate (Pearlin and Schooler, 1978; Folkman and Lazarus, 1980). It makes the situation comprehensible, connecting the present with the past and the future. It merges life's events into a flow.

Thus there are two characteristic attributions that I have identified here whose presence indicates the lack of a sense of cognitive coherence: fatalism and meaninglessness. The coherence hypothesis, that religion benefits health because it promotes a sense of coherence in individuals, can now be sharpened by hypothesizing that religious interpretations diminish attributions of fatalism and/or meaninglessness. It is thus the interpretive, reflective, and subjective aspects of religious involvement that are of interest here, in contrast to the public, participatory social activities of the cohesiveness hypothesis.

The *coherence hypothesis* states that the relationship between religious involvement and health is explained by the sense of cognitive coherence provided by religious interpretations of life situations.

It may be important to point out that there is no either-or agenda in mind here. Religious involvement has both a cognitive and a social reality for individuals. It can be fruitfully understood in both a Durkheimian and a Weberian manner. Neither reality is more true than the other, though one or the other may indeed be more relevant to health. Moreover, given the length of the possible causal chains involved, it may be neither the cohesiveness nor the coherence hypothesis, but the behavioral hypothesis that is most likely to be supported by the data. In any case, the relevance of all three intervening hypotheses to both health and religion has been demonstrated, and hence the importance of considering them. These hypotheses have been proposed thus far at the most general level, but as they are they represent a more developed theoretical approach to the epidemiology of religion than has heretofore appeared. There are some previous studies whose findings are important, however, and with these we conclude the chapter.

The Epidemiology of Religion

Truly only a handful of epidemiological studies have considered the role of religious involvement, in any form whatever, in association with health, measured in any way whatever. Study designs range from major long-term follow-up studies (Berkman and Syme, 1979; House, Robbins, and Metzner, 1982) to small, non-random-sample cross-sectional measurements (Ness, 1980). The measurements of health have also varied from several indicators of mental health all the way to mortality. For these reasons, most of the studies are, for all practical purposes, not comparable (except where noted). What does not change much from one study to the other is the measure of religion used: it is almost always limited to a unidimensional measure, either church membership or church attendance.

All-Cause Mortality Studies

By far the most striking studies are the longitudinal studies which have mortality outcomes (Blazer and Palmore, 1976; Comstock and Tonascia, 1977; Berkman and Syme, 1979; Wingard, 1982; House, Robbins, and Metzner, 1982; Reed, McGee and Yano, 1984; Zuckerman, Kasl, and Ostfeld, 1984).

In the largest of the studies, Comstock and Partridge (1972) and Comstock and Tonascia (1977) analyzed data including church attendance from a 1963 complete census of Washington County, Maryland, and an 8-year follow-up of death records. Admittedly without a theory in mind, (1972, p. 668) they found higher death rates for the 8-year period at each of five levels of decreasing church attendance. On closer examination, however (1977), they discovered that the inverse association of church attendance and mortality was strongest during the early years of the follow-up and disappeared in the last two years. Their interpretation was that a selection effect was operating, and that church attendance was primarily serving as a measure of functional status. The authors were unable to control for health status at the beginning of the study, since no measure of health status or functional ability was included in the 1963 survey.

The second study was done in Alameda County, California, in a 1974 follow-up of 1965 data from a random sample of 6928 adults (Berkman and Syme, 1979). The importance of this study was not its findings regarding the decreased mortality risk for church members specifically, but its demonstration of increased mortality risk for people who lacked social and community ties in general. The men and women found to be most socially isolated in 1965 were between two and three times as likely to die in the follow-up period as those with the most social ties. The key finding of the study was that the association between mortality and the lack of social ties was independent of numerous better-known risk factors, including socioeconomic status, the poor health practices of smoking, drinking, obesity, and physical inactivity, and importantly, health status at the beginning of the follow-up period. The four types of social contact presciently included in the 1965 survey were: 1) marriage, 2) contacts with close friends and relatives, 3) church or temple congregation membership, and 4) informal and formal group associations. By and large, each of these four sources of social contact was associated with lower mortality rates, although marriage seemed to make no difference to women and group membership had no effect for men. But regardless of age or sex, individuals who belonged to a religious group had significantly lower mortality rates during the follow-up period than those who did not.

Wingard's (1982) reanalysis of the Alameda County data was undertaken to explain the sex differential in mortality rates. She found, as did Berkman and Syme, that men were less likely to be church or temple members than women, and that the age-adjusted mortality rates for members (men and women) were significantly lower than for nonmembers. When a full range of demographic, health behavior, social behavior, and psychological variables were entered, however, the relationship between church or temple membership and mortality disappeared. The discrepancy between this finding and that of Berkman and Syme is explained by their use of a social network index and Wingard's analysis of the components. Berkman and Syme did not report results of controlling for health status or health practices in the analysis of the individual social ties. It is harder to argue for a selection effect in the Alameda County studies, though, when the measure was of religious group *membership*, rather than *attendance*.

The fourth major longitudinal study was conducted in Tecumseh County, Michigan, with a twelve-year follow-up of a cohort of 2754 adult men and women (House, Robbins, and Metzner, 1982). The range of social relationships and activities examined in this study was much broader than in Alameda County, but less conceptually precise. The intent was to assess the effects on mortality of the frequency of, and satisfaction with social participation, as well as the types of existing relationships. For men, the results were rather similar to the Berkman and Syme study: the more actively involved men were in social relationships and activities, the less likely they were to die in the follow-up period. After adjusting for age and other risk factors, the social relationships/activities of marriage, attending association meetings, spectator events, and lectures continued to predict lower mortality rates. Frequency of religious service attendance did not predict mortality for men, either before or after adjustment for risk factors. For women, however, attendance at religious services was the only social relationship/activity which was associated with lower mortality rates when the risk factors were controlled. Several social factors which had zero-order associations, marriage, frequency of going on outings, and attending spectator events, lost significance after adjustments, but church attendance actually increased in significance, indicating the existence of some suppression effect. The authors suggest that some of the differences in "processes of social integration and activity" between rural, midwestern Tecumseh County and urban, heterogeneous Alameda County may have been responsible for the differences in results.

The final published study with mortality rate as the health outcome is a two-year follow-up study of 400 elderly people in Connecticut (Zuckerman, Kasl, and Ostfeld, 1984). Originally a study of the health effects of residential relocation, data collection also included information on social contacts, feelings of well-being, and three forms of religious involvement. An index of religiousness was created by summing the scores for three questions, "How often did you attend regular religious services during the year?", "Aside from how often you attended regular religious services, do you consider yourself to be deeply religious, fairly religious, only slightly religious, not at all religious, or against religion?", and "How much is religion a source of strength and comfort to you?"[4] Each of the items had a significant, inverse association with mortality at the two-year follow-up; church attendance less strongly so, getting strength from religion more strongly. When demographic factors, relocation, and health status at the beginning of the follow-up were controlled, the index of religiousness had no significant main effect on mortality. In interaction with the health index, however, it was a highly significant predictor of mortality. The protective effect of religiousness is evident only among the elderly in poor health, both among the men and the women. The elderly in poor health who were less religious were twice as likely to die in the two-year follow-up period as those in poor health who were more religious. This is very important because it suggests that previous studies which failed to find a main effect of religion after controlling for health status might well have found a significant interaction. On the other hand, perhaps this is only true for the elderly. This study is unique in several ways which make it very relevant to the present study: it underscores the need for more manifold measures of religious involvement tapping private perceptions as well as public behaviors, and it begins to indicate the complexity of the relationship between religion and the health of the elderly.

Disease-Specific Studies

The studies in this category are more numerous, though few are so well-designed as the best of those above. As long ago as the 1950's epidemiologists were aware of the lower prevalence of cancer and coronary heart disease among Seventh-Day Adventists. One analysis of the records of eight Seventh-Day Adventist hospitals showed significantly lower incidences of cancers of the lung, mouth, larynx, esophagus, bladder (men), and cervix (women) (Wynder, Lemon, and Bross, 1959). Another early study compared rates of hypertension and coronary heart disease among Trappist and Benedictine monks in Belgium and the Netherlands (Groen et al., 1962). Although they found no difference in the prevalence of myocardial infarctions between them, the two orders had much lower rates than the rest of the population. A third imaginative early study compared the hypertension rates of South African Zulu who had migrated to urban areas, with those who had remained in a tribal area. Although this was true only for women, in both the city and the reserve, church membership or attendance was associated with normal blood pressure (Scotch, 1963). For men it was quite different: church attendance in the reserve was associated with lower blood pressure, but in the city, church membership was associated with *higher* blood pressure. Scotch observes that church membership is deviant for men in the city, thus it is not the "healthy outlet" that it is for women.

More recent studies have focused on the relationship between religion and diseases of the cardiovascular system. Jenkins' early (1971) review of the psychological and social precursors of coronary heart disease found few epidemiologic studies that "tabulated" religion. The seven studies he mentions are all concerned with religious preference differences and coronary heart disease. Few consistent findings emerge; some find higher rates among Protestants, some among Jews. In addition to their mortality data, Comstock and Partridge report inverse associations of church attendance and five-year incidence rates for tuberculosis and prevalence ratios (among women) for trichomoniasis and abnormal cervical cytology, findings which may not be subject to the same selection effects. Another study of coronary heart disease, this of three-year incidence rates for myocardial infarction, found the more religious among 10,000 male Israeli government employees to have lower rates of myocardial infarction than the less religious (Medalie et al., 1973). The Evans County

Cardiovascular Epidemiologic Study (Graham et al., 1978) reported a cross-sectional association between blood pressure and church attendance for white males. Both systolic and diastolic blood pressures were lower among frequent church attenders than among infrequent attenders, a relationship that persisted even when age, obesity, smoking, and socioeconomic status were controlled.

Most recently, Hannay (1980) found a cross-sectional association of active religious participation and lower scores on a 44-item checklist of physical symptoms suffered during the previous two weeks. The study sample was randomly selected from the registry of a health center in Glasgow, Scotland (N=964). And in an attempt to explain the well-known lower cancer incidence rates of Mormons in Utah, church members were stratified by position and activity level in the church, presumably an indication of their adherence to church doctrine, some aspects of which are known to be health-related (Gardner and Lyon, 1982a; Gardner and Lyon, 1982b). Among men, the most devout (classified by lay priesthood office) were found to have lung cancer rates 80 percent lower than that of the least devout group. Cancer of the stomach, leukemias, lymphomas, and all smoking- and alcohol-related cancer sites were all least frequent in the most devout group (Gardner and Lyon, 1982a). Mormon women with the strongest adherence to church doctrine had significantly lower lung cancer rates, but the study found no differences for breast, ovarian, or gastrointestinal cancers (Gardner and Lyon, 1982b).

These studies indicate the possibility of a connection between religious involvement of one kind or another with several types of serious illness and with death from all causes. But there are relatively few studies, and attempts at theoretical explanation are so rudimentary, if not nonexistent, that the field must be considered barely surveyed.

Mental Illness Studies

The earliest epidemiological studies of religion and mental illness focused on the differing rates and types of disorder found among Protestants, Catholics, and Jews. In a study of the psychiatric in-treatment population in New Haven, Roberts and Myers (1954) found Catholics to have more than the expected number of diagnoses of alcohol and drug addiction, and Jews more than the expected number of psychoneurotic disorders. In another New Haven study, Hollingshead and Redlich (1958) (who were interested in religion only as it modified the effects of social class on mental illness) found Protestants in the lowest social class to be about two and a half times more likely than expected to be in treatment. In the Midtown Manhattan Study, a random sample of households revealed significantly more impairment among Jews than among Protestants or Catholics; and the highest rates of inpatient hospital treatment for Catholics (Srole et al., 1977 [1962]). Another early study took a communitarian religious sect, the Hutterites, as its epidemiological laboratory, enumerating all forms of mental illness in the population (Eaton and Weil, 1955). While they found no lack of mental illness, they concluded that Hutterite mental patients reflected Hutterite culture in their symptoms. I am aware of only four studies that have attempted to correlate some measure of mental health with religious involvement rather than with nominal affiliation. Curiously, the Midtown Study asked about their respondents' parents' commitment to their faith, but not that of the respondents themselves. They found the most favorable mental health among those respondents whose parents were in the middle range, to whom religion was somewhat important, and the worst among those whose parents thought religion not important at all (Srole et al., 1977 [1962]). Gurin, Veroff, and Feld (1960) reported a tendency for infrequently-attending Catholics to admit more worry, less happiness, and more feelings of distress than Catholics who went to church regularly, but these were not strong relationships. A cross-sectional study of impairment, church attendance, and prayer found that among the most impaired, proportionately fewer attended church regularly, but more prayed, especially in response to certain life events (Lindenthal et al., 1970). An ethnographic epidemiological study in Newfoundland compared the health and religious involvement of members of two small rural churches, one Pentecostal and the other mainline Protestant (Ness, 1980). The author found increased religious ritual participation to be associated with fewer psychological complaints on the Cornell Medical Index, but this was true only in the more closely-knit Pentecostal Church.

Thus there are even fewer studies of mental health and religious involvement than there are of physical health. Furthermore, the existence of a correlation between religious involvement and psychological distress is not always confirmed, the direction of the relationship is questionable (the Lindenthal et al. study found frequency of prayer *positively* associated with impairment), and no two studies are even remotely comparable, given their differing measurements of both distress and religious involvement. All in all, little or nothing is known about the relationship of religious involvement and mental health.

There is a great deal to be learned from this recitation of study results. In general, one would have to say that a number of these studies are methodologically very well-designed and executed, with large populations, long follow-up periods, careful analysis and reanalysis. The important methodological issues are well-understood, and the ways to make future studies better are fairly clear. What is almost completely lacking, however, is a well-grounded theoretical understanding of religion, some basis on which one might be able to say *why* religion does or does not have a relationship to health. The few theories that there are, and these are more implicit than explicit, see religion as the promoter of certain good health practices, or as the location of social network interaction. There is no attention at all to the content and substance of religion. Even a cross-sectional study could make progress in this area. This lack of theory is precisely what is responsible for the biggest methodological weakness in these studies: the measurement of the concept itself. A simple yes/no answer to whether or not one is a church member is not sufficient. With a more adequate theoretical grasp of what religion is, however, one can deconstruct the considerable complexity of religious involvement. At a very minimum, and above all in studies of the elderly, one must distinguish the active, service-attending aspects of religious involvement that require physical mobility from the private, reflective aspects that require nothing but consciousness.

Future studies should also contain a wider variety of health measurements, with more emphasis on morbidity since that is where least is known. Utilizing a range of health measures, including both highly objective and highly subjective indicators could also be very informative. These, then, could form the basis for the means of controlling for health status. Controls for objective physical health status are as important in a cross-sectional study as they are in follow-up, though perhaps not easy to specify. Controlling for the more objective, physical measures while looking at the more subjective measures seems a logical way to proceed.

In the end, the most convincing conclusion will come from proposing, developing, and testing theoretically sound explanations for the hypothesized positive effect of religion on health. This chapter has endeavored to sketch out what some of those mediating relationships might be, and their relevance to the classical theory traditions in the sociology of religion. The behavioral, cohesiveness, and coherence hypotheses are all plausible reasons why religion may have some positive effect on health. In the language of data analysis, these are the arguments for the main and indirect effects of religion. In the next chapter an alternative is considered, the possibility that religion modifies the impact of physical health on an individual's psychological distress and subjective perceptions of health. This is the fourth and final explanatory hypothesis, the theodicy hypothesis.

Notes to Chapter I

[1]This is not the place to discuss the Protestant Ethic thesis controversy, although a brief word should be said about Weber's understanding of causality. It was Weber's belief, and his intent in writing the *Protestant Ethic and Spirit of Capitalism* to show that religious values freely chosen, were able to influence economic behavior and create a context which encouraged a new attitude to work and wealth and within which that attitude became intelligible. If the Protestant Ethic seems limited to an explanation of one half of a dialectical relationship, that religious beliefs only caused economic behaviors and were not affected by them, it is because Weber correctly surmised that Marx had compellingly enough shown the argument for the other causal direction, the importance of which Weber never denied.

[2]The names are used by Gottlieb (1981) but I have changed the meanings.

[3]His acknowledgement (p. 179).

[4]These items are virtually identical to three used in the Yale Health and Aging Project and the present study.

II
Religion at the Boundaries: Aging and Illness

. . . man is born to trouble
   as the sparks fly upward. (Job 5:7)

Therefore let everyone who is godly
   offer prayer to thee;
at a time of distress, in the rush of great waters,
   they shall not reach him.
Thou art a hiding place for me,
   thou preservest me from trouble;
   thou dost encompass me with deliverance.

I will instruct you and teach you
   the way you should go;
I will counsel you with my eye upon you.
   Be not like a horse or a mule,
   without understanding. (Psalm 32:6-9)

Even though I walk through the
   valley of the shadow of death,
   I fear no evil;
for thou art with me;
   thy rod and thy staff
   they comfort me. (Psalm 23:4)

In Chapter I, the theoretical reasons for a direct association of religious involvement and health were outlined, and several plausible mechanisms through which religion may be indirectly associated with health were hypothesized. In Chapter II we raise the further possibility that an individual's religious involvement may interact in some way with his or her state of health, in other words, that religious involvement may have differing consequences for the well and ill

39

elderly. This is the fourth and final explanatory hypothesis: the theodicy hypothesis. The direction of the predicted association is the same, again the relationship should be positive. The difference is that effects of religious involvement are predicted to be stronger for certain disadvantaged groups.

The findings of the Zuckerman, Kasl, and Ostfeld (1984) study reported in the first chapter underscore the importance of testing for such an interaction effect. In that study, there was only a modest effect of religious involvement in predicting mortality, and if the authors had failed to test for an interaction effect, their conclusion would have been that religiosity played little role in the health of that elderly population. Their results, however, showed that religiosity significantly decreased the risk of mortality among precisely those at highest risk: the elderly in poor health.

The present study, of course, does not have the methodological advantage of follow-up data on mortality, and thus no way to test for an interaction of religious involvement and morbidity in predicting mortality. What it does have, however, has its own advantages: a range of measures of morbidity, disabling consequences of morbidity, perceptions of morbidity, and psychological distress. It will thus be possible, not only to look at, for example, the relationship of religiousness and functional disability while holding constant the level of chronic conditions, but also to test for the interaction between religiousness and chronic conditions.

There are substantial theoretical reasons for expecting to find religiousness particularly relevant to the elderly in poor health. Both classical sociological theories of religion and contemporary findings in social psychological research form a basis for anticipating that religious involvement may be especially salient in situations of suffering or tragic events.

The Theodicy Hypothesis

When confronted with permanent and unchangeable circumstances people are forced to cope, however well or poorly. When these circumstances are threatening, or when they portend uncertainty, the importance of coping increases. When the things one values most--the life, health, and security of oneself and loved ones--are threatened, the circumstances become existentially critical. These situations, often called "boundary situations" become the points of articulation between human experience and religious cosmology. Illness, bereavement, fear, guilt, deprivation, all strip away the taken-for-granted character of daily life and force consideration of one's ultimate values. They are the foxholes that open up under one's feet, recalling the ultimate impermanence of life. Bakan (1968) has argued that in experiences of suffering, pain can be coped with in two ways: either suffering can be wiped out by oblivion, or it can be enhanced through understanding. Pain and threat press for interpretation. The fact that many people seek religion at moments of crisis is not so much a commentary on human complacency and hypocrisy as it is a sure indication that religion has something to offer in those situations. Religion is, according to John Bowker (1973), the "way through" the intransigencies of human existence. As a cognitive map, it provides assurance that there is a route, that it can be found, and even that one's progress along it can be gauged. This is not to say that religion provides direction less in noncrisis situations, but only that the reasons for its evident salience in situations of suffering are anthropologically sound.

Historically, the explanations that religions have provided for human suffering have been called theodicies, from the Greek *theos*, meaning 'god' and *dike*, meaning 'justice,' "a writing, doctrine, or theory intended to 'justify the ways of God to men'" (Shorter Oxford English Dictionary). The problem of "justifying God's ways" becomes necessary when the god is seen as a good god who is powerful enough to intervene in human affairs. In a classic statement of the problem, Bowker (1970) writes,

> . . . if God is all-loving he would surely not be able to tolerate the appalling suffering that is evident in the created order; and if he is almighty, he would be able to do something about it (p. 81).

Given the existence of good and evil in the world, the question is not so much why suffering exists but why it is dealt out the way it is:

. . . he destroys both the blameless and the wicked (Job 9:22).

How can a righteous god allow the innocent to suffer? Weber (1922) noted that karma, in which life is seen as a never-ending wheel of reward and retribution, and Calvinism, in which all human events are predestined and controlled by God, are the two most consistent theodicies. He grouped theodicies of the world religions into five types: the sufferer will be compensated for his suffering in this world through a revolutionary change in social conditions; or the sufferer will be compensated after death with a reward in heaven; or good and evil can be seen as locked in continual dualistic struggle; or good and evil can be relativized by karma, the turning wheel of fate; or the reality of suffering can be somehow negated through metempsychosis. Weber's typology has been criticized by Geertz (1973) for being too intellectual and not attending to the affective aspect of meaning, of making suffering sufferable. Berger (1967) has elaborated Weber's typology noting that underlying all theodicies there is a basic surrender of the self to some larger order. A theodicy, as the resolution of a paradox, is both a means for assigning cause and an assurance that an order exists.

In the contemporary language of attribution theory, when the individual is confronted with a permanent, nonmodifiable outcome (Wortman and Brehm, 1975), or an aversive situation in which the attribution of fatalism is a reflection of the individual's true helplessness, the attribution of meaning given by theodicies would be of special importance. In fact, if it were not a contradiction in terms, attributions could be thought of as "agnostic theodicies," a class of explanations for suffering that would subsume religious theodicies. Indeed, attributions of meaning from the secular psychological standpoint are sometimes seen as functionally equivalent alternatives to religion (Luckmann, 1967), although Ernest Becker's *The Denial of Death* is a passionate argument against this position (1973). The relative adequacy of religious and non-religious explanations for suffering is in some sense an empirical question though it has never been studied; a recent article on theodicies in bereavement notes that empirical studies of theodicies are rare (Wuthnow, Christiano, and Kuzlowski, 1980). But religious or not, the attribution of meaning must be based on a shared belief system if it is to be accessible to social-psychological analysis.

Shared religious belief systems, as opposed to self-generated, idiosyncratic ones, merge the believer's identity with a larger group.

In the case of the major world religions, these "groups" cut across cultures and back through historical time. They thus not only join the believer to an immediate, present society capable of delivering tangible social support, but also to the historical collectivity of believers, both living and dead. The life of the collective is easily seen as stretching back through time and on into the future, well beyond the individual's life span. Individual believers, then, participate in the immortality of the collective in all historical religions, regardless of their beliefs about individual immortality (Bakan, 1968). Group worship and ritual, in this connection, serve the purpose of fusing individual and collective fate by bringing social structure to consciousness (Turner, 1969). The more frequent the group activity, the more enhanced this consciousness of a sort of spiritual cohesiveness, and the more easily it can be called on as a way through the boundary situations that threaten earthly life.

Events of illness and physical suffering have occupied an important place in the Judeo-Christian tradition from the fall of man. The biblical tradition addressing the cognitive problem arising from the experience of personal suffering begins with Job. Thus the possibilities for attributing religious meaning to problems of physical suffering and mortality are available, well-elaborated, and plausible. They are not, however, particularly systematic or logical, as has often been pointed out (Bowker, 1970). It is not the explanation of the suffering *per se* that is important, but the belief in the explanation; indeed a belief system's lack of internal interrelatedness can actually protect its overall integrity (Snow and Machalek, 1982).

A definitive categorization of theodicies of personal suffering must await further empirical study. Wuthnow, Christiano, and Kuzlowski, (1980) have proposed a typology for theodicies of bereavement based on blaming God, the self, life, the mind, or the imagination. A reading of contemporary religious writing on illness may suggest some others (Vaux, 1978; Lewis, 1962; Kelsey, 1973).

-Illness and suffering may be seen as punishment for sins committed, God's way of calling for repentance.

-Illness and suffering may be seen as a test of the strength of faith.

-Illness and suffering may be seen as the cause of a conversion or a renewed religious experience.

-Suffering may be seen as exemplary and ennobling.

-The causes of illness and suffering may be seen as beyond human comprehension, an indication of God's omniscience.

-Suffering can be seen as sacrificial, as being for the good of others.

All of these Judeo-Christian ways of thinking about personal suffering have one thing in common pointed out earlier in connection with theodicies in general: they have the effect of submerging the individual in something larger than the self, and are all in that way masochistic (Berger, 1967). The self is, so to speak, given up. The sense of surrender to the Other, in fact, is the core of the religious experience. Classic writings on the nature of the religious experience (Otto, 1917; James, 1901-1902) have emphasized the universality of the feelings of religious experience--the cognizance of and submersion in a power and reality greater than one's own.

Thus the religious experience itself may contain some elements of helplessness. So is it possible that religious beliefs foster feelings of hopefulness independently of feelings of helplessness? Does the ability to give religious meaning to situations of personal suffering condition the very different kinds of individual reactions to life crises that are frequently noted by investigators (Silver and Wortman, 1980)? Silver and Wortman (1980) in fact, call for a study of "variables that may mediate individual coping responses" which are "necessary to explain the diverse pattern of results" (p. 309). The mediating variables they suggest incorporating include: social support, the opportunity for free expression of feelings, the ability to find meaning in the crisis, or experience with other stressors (p. 326). Their review of the few existing empirical studies suggests that "the ability to find meaning may be important" (p. 318). The observation they do not make is that the meanings they give as examples are most often religious.

Coping researchers have been hard pressed to explain the paradoxical finding that religious individuals blame themselves for their own or their child's illness and at the same time seem to cope better. Given that the tendency for people to assign blame increases as the magnitude of the misfortune increases (Walster, 1966), and that self-blame entails greater illusion of control than blaming external forces (Wortman and Brehm, 1975), the association of self-blame with serious illness or disability is perhaps predictable. The question is, why should religious individuals be more likely than the non-religious to blame themselves? In a study of victims of severe accidents, Bulman and Wortman (1977) found the very religious significantly more likely to blame themselves, and that overall, the more a victim blamed him or herself, regardless of the objective evidence, the better they coped. The majority of the victims' ascriptions of meaning carried manifest religious content. Bulman and Wortman (1977) note that their respondents were very concerned with justice, and this may provide the solution to the puzzle: religion in the form of a theodicy at once provides the means for assigning moral blame, and the means for its removal. If the cause of misfortune can be attributed to sin or human finitude, religious repentance and forgiveness are always available as resolution.

In situations of helplessness where blame is less relevant, such as in illness, religious interpretations may promote acceptance of difficult situations if they are deemed spiritually meaningful. Recent research on depression and coping in stressful episodes has shown that depressed people are less likely to have "accepted" their situation (Coyne, Aldwin, and Lazarus, 1981). They were also significantly more likely to brood over their problems saying they needed more information, to wish they were stronger, and that they could change the way they felt. If the "acceptance" of a situation depends on having a cognitively and emotionally satisfying interpretation of it, that would explain why the depressed subjects in this study appeared so uncertain. They had obviously not constructed a coherent "acceptable" account of their situation. That religion promotes such acceptance is the conclusion of a British physician examining a recent group of pilgrims to Lourdes (Morris, 1982). He noted that while their physical condition on the whole was not improved, they were significantly less depressed on their return, and felt that "the visit had been beneficial, in that it had strengthened their religious faith, and had made them more relaxed, more content and more able to accept their physical disabilities" (p. 294). The suggestion in both of these studies is that it is not only interpretations of the situation that are at issue here, but interpretations of the self that also make a difference. One may learn things about oneself in suffering, and one's view of oneself may change. This was precisely the finding of the famous worm-eating study (Comer and Laird, 1975). They found that students who anticipated an unpleasant task made sense of it to themselves in such a way that they then actually chose to suffer when it was no longer mandatory. This view of suffering as formative of the self suggests that the attribution of meaning in a specific situation of suffering is very likely to form, or to reflect an already-formed characteristic, generalized attribution of meaning or meaninglessness.

The importance of attributions of meaning in situations of true helplessness is perfectly summed up by Reinhold Niebuhr in a prayer which Alcoholics Anonymous has made familiar:

> Oh God, give us the serenity to accept what cannot be changed, courage to change what should be changed, and wisdom to distinguish the one from the other (quoted in Wortman and Brehm, 1975, pp. 331-332).

Acceptance of one's helplessness extends ultimately to the awareness of one's mortality, which William James (1901-1902) called "the worm at the core." One might think that those closest to death, the very elderly, would be likely to fear it most. But while the elderly apparently do think about death more than the young, they also fear it less, having reached some acceptance of it (Jeffers and Verwoerdt, 1969; Kalish and Reynolds, 1976; Kalish and Johnson, 1972; Lieberman and Coplan, 1970).

One might also think that the more religious would be least afraid of death, but again the evidence is contradictory. While a few, mostly older studies, have shown religious beliefs to be associated with lower death anxiety (Feifel and Branscomb, 1973; Swenson, 1961; Williams and Cole, 1968; Martin and Wrightsman, 1965), and other studies have been inconclusive or shown no relationship (Lester, 1967; Templer, 1972), the most interesting studies have shown religion to have a curvilinear relationship with the fear of death, with the most deeply religious and a small but important group at the other end, the most adamantly non-religious, having the least fear of death (Kalish and Reynolds, 1976; Templer and Dotson, 1970; McMordie, 1981; Kubler-Ross, 1969). Kalish and Reynolds (1976), weighing the results of their survey of attitudes toward death among four Los Angeles ethnic groups (N=434), comment,

> Who fears death the most? Our answer must be: those who lack a reasonably firm acceptance of some coherent life system that tries to make death understandable and that tries to make life meaningful. We feel, therefore, with

Kubler-Ross, that the firmly devout and the true non-believers can cope with death more effectively than those whose views are vague or ambivalent (p.91).

When they examined the elderly alone, however, they found very few elderly among the group of "true non-believers." Thus among young and middle-aged adults it is the presence of a "coherent life system" and not religion *per se* that is associated with the attribution of meaning to life, even in the situation of universal helplessness. But among the elderly, the more likely pattern appears to be a religious, rather than a "true non-believing" source of meaning.

Serious chronic illness is one of the most crucial of the boundary situations, a primary example of a situation of true helplessness. An examination of the religious involvement of the elderly in these situations and their attributions of fatalism and/or meaning may aid the development of the still-embryonic empirical study of theodicies. The theodicy hypothesis, in a word, is that religious involvement will lessen the distress an individual feels when suffering serious illness or disability.

The *theodicy hypothesis* states that, in objective conditions of illness or disability, higher levels of religious involvement will be associated with lower subjective perceptions of suffering.

The Religious Involvement of the Aging

Do people become more religious as they age? Common sense urges a positive answer; the stereotype of piety in old age is highly believable. Research on religious participation throughout the lifespan, however, has not shown dramatic changes in religiosity with age. Instead, a well-known article by Bahr (1970) proposes four models for describing the relationship between church attendance and age, none of which predict sharply increased religiosity for the aged: 1) a traditional model, in which teenagers' high level of attendance drops to a life-cycle low in the early thirties and then climbs steadily into old age; 2) a lifetime stability model, in which there is little change; 3) a family life-cycle model, in which the peak in attendance coincides with the child-rearing period; and 4) a disengagement model, which focuses on the declining attendance of the elderly. Each model has some empirical work to support it (Fichter, 1952; Glock, Ringer and Babbie, 1967; Lazerwitz, 1961; Orbach, 1961; Riley and Foner, 1968; Argyle, 1958), but each suffers from being based on analysis of cross-sectional or retrospective data, making age effects impossible to differentiate from cohort effects. This entanglement is revealed by Orbach's (1961) finding of increased attendance among older Jews, not an age effect at all, but an artifact of the historic decline of orthodox Judaism in this country. Only a cohort analysis can determine whether changes in church attendance should be attributed to aging or to history. Wingrove and Alston's (1974) analysis of national survey data on the church attendance of six ten-year cohorts showed that both are probably involved: they found as many differences in attendance *between* generations as *within* them.

On the other hand, the elderly are far more likely than other age groups to say they have no doubt that there is a life after death (Stark, 1968; Cavan et al., 1949; Kalish and Reynolds, 1976); to turn to their clergyman for comfort (Kalish and Reynolds, 1976); to be the most highly orthodox in their belief (Stark, 1968); to perform private devotions (Stark, 1968); and to have a religiously-optimistic outlook (McCready and Greeley, 1976). These findings, again, may be the result of cohort and not age effects, but the immediate conclusion to be drawn is that any discussion of religion and aging must carefully distinguish the public, ritual participation aspects from private devotional activities and religious belief.

Looking at the aged themselves as a group, nearly every study reports some decline in church attendance among the very elderly, though in some it does not begin until very late, and the decline is less than for any other voluntary organization (Moberg, 1965; Cutler, 1976). Those few studies (Heenan, 1972) that have looked at both public and private religious activity, however, have inevitably contrasted the decline in the former with the persistence of the latter, and cited physical infirmity, rather than lack of interest, as the cause (Palmore, 1969; Moberg, 1965). As long ago as 1949, Cavan et al., observed that in their sample the private religious activities of listening to church services on the radio and reading the Bible increased, and more than compensated for any decline in church attendance. Fukuyama's (1961) survey of 4095 Congregational Church members, using Glock and Stark's (1965) multiple dimensions of religiosity, showed older members to be more religious creedally and devotionally, but less involved in public worship services. Stark's own study (1968) of 2871 San Francisco area church members showed a great increase in private devotionalism with age among both Roman Catholics and Protestants, along with an increase in public ritual involvement among Protestants, but not Catholics, over age 70.

The authors of a study of 106 elderly Missourians argue specifically that the failure to consider nonorganizational forms of religiosity has fostered the misconception that the elderly are religiously "disengaged" (Mindel and Vaughan, 1978; see Cumming and Henry, 1961; and Hochschild, 1975). They found their infrequent church attenders to engage in nonorganizational religious activities (listening to services on radio or TV, praying, listening to religious music, feeling that religion has helped in understanding life) slightly *more* often than the frequent attenders. Moreover, a measure of physical impairment was not related to organizational involvement, but the more impaired elderly did engage in more nonorganizational religious activities. Steinitz' (1978) analysis of NORC data (N = 1493) goes a step further and considers the effect of health and church attendance on a general measure of well-being, concluding that the relationship between church attendance and well-being depends on the health of the elderly:

> Apparently, if frail elderly persons overcome their health limitations sufficiently to attend religious services, they experience considerable happiness, excitement, and satisfaction in their lives. But regular attendance makes little difference to the well-being of healthy older people (p. 62).

Overall, she found a belief in life after death to be more strongly associated with well-being than was church attendance.

With regard to more precise health measures, this public/private dimension of the elderly's religiosity has only twice been assessed, to my knowledge. Blazer and Palmore (1976), reporting on 20-year follow-up data from the well-known Duke Longitudinal Study, found their 272 volunteers to decrease their religious activity over time, but to maintain a very constant level of religious attitudes. They found no relationship between longevity and either religious activities or religious attitudes, but both activities and attitudes were strongly correlated with feelings of happiness. The other study is the Zuckerman, Kasl, and Ostfeld (1984) study discussed earlier, in which the measure of religiousness combined religious attitudes and activities.

They found religiousness to predict survival among the elderly only among the less healthy, and religious attitudes to be more strongly predictive of survival than religious activities. These findings are especially notable in view of the House, Robbins, and Metzner (1982) finding that *non*-religious solitary pastimes such as watching TV or reading were associated with an *increase* in mortality.

One could sum up the findings of the studies of religion and aging by saying that there is no dramatic change in religious involvement as individuals become elderly. The type of involvement most likely to diminish with age is public attendance at religious services, most often for health reasons. There is no evidence at all for a decline in private forms of religious involvements which may, in fact, increase.

The Religious Involvement of Women

Surely the most enduring finding in the scientific study of religion is that women, young and old, married and unmarried, are more involved than men in religious activities. In 1950 Gordon Allport could write with certainty,

> It is common in all studies to find women more interested in religion however defined. They are more often the church-goers, more often devout in their personal lives, and more often the family mentors in matters of religion (Allport, 1950, p. 37).

Individual studies have found women more religious than men in the cultic, creedal, and devotional senses (Fukuyama, 1961); more ritualistic, altruistic, fundamentalistic, theistic, idealistic, superstitious, and mystical (Maranell, 1974). National survey data have shown women to be especially overrepresented in the membership of the Episcopalian and black Baptist churches (Lazerwitz, 1961), while older white Catholic women have been found to be the most frequent church-attenders, both nationally (Alston and McIntosh, 1979), and in a Detroit area study (Orbach, 1961). Wingrove and Alston's (1974) cohort analysis, when broken down by sex, graphically demonstrates women's historically higher church attendance levels, both inter- and intra-generationally. Studies that have restricted themselves to the church attendance patterns of the elderly have reported similar findings

(Cavan et al., 1949; Maves, 1960; Gray and Moberg, 1962; Riley and Foner, 1968). The Duke Longitudinal Study (Blazer and Palmore, 1976), found their elderly black and white women to be significantly more religious than the men, in both attitude and activity. Heisel and Faulkner (1982) found black women's religiosity significantly exceeding men's *only* among the elderly.

But this relationship has more often been observed than analyzed. In not one of the above-mentioned studies, in fact, is any explanation at all offered, other than to note that this is what studies always find. Argyle (1958) offers a psychoanalytic argument that women have more guilt feelings than men and that on the basis of parent-child, opposite-sex attraction, are more likely to be drawn to a projected father-figure God. A sort of psychological compensation theory is proposed by Komarovsky, whose unhappy blue-collar wives drew on religion for "psychological strength" (1962, p. 124).

Sociological explanations have dwelt on religion's (and women's) role in the transmission of social values and roles. A classical statement of this theoretical approach can be found in Fichter, who initially dismisses the "psychological suggestion" that women are "naturally" more pious. Rather,

> . . . the religious role is more compatible with the other roles of women than with the other roles of men. For example, both their roles in the family and as culture-bearers in this society imply functions and values which are relatively consistent with the functions and values of religion. Women are still supposed to promote and exemplify the 'higher things of life'. On the other hand, the secular roles (occupational, political, recreational, and so forth) of the male are more likely to be in conflict with his religious role (1952, p. 149).

In other words, women are more religious than men because they bear both the culture and the next generation and because they experience less role conflict with religion than men do. Other versions of this argument can be found in Lenski (1953) who concentrated on the role conflict strand, and Glock et al. (1967), who emphasized the socializing function of religious values. Noting that the contemporary church is not "reasserting its historical authority in the economic realm" (p. 44), they see women as more motivated toward religious involvement and having more opportunity for it. If this were true, however, one would expect some historical changes showing up in the cohort analysis discussed earlier (Wingrove and Alston, 1974), but there are none which do not affect men and women in approximately the same way. Closer analysis by changes in gender roles should clarify the issues.

The functionalist implication of this argument is that women are necessary for the transmission of the complex of religious and social values to children, and thus that religion is a conservative force in maintaining traditional gender roles. Historically, however, and in spite of its patriarchal reputation, it has recently been argued that Western Christianity has been a force for changes in gender relations, especially in the period of early Christianity and at the Reformation (Elshtain, 1981). A recent study of women's religious service attendance patterns and their move into the work force concludes that women who work *are* less likely to attend church services, but that both working and church attendance are the products of a woman's predisposing personal characteristics (Ulbrich and Wallace, 1984).

In any case, these explanations are less helpful in discussing the religious involvement of the elderly. While older men's and women's social roles become more similar their religious involvement diverges. Are there differences in the meaning of religion for elderly men and women? For one thing, if religious involvement is more normative for elderly women than it is for men, as all the data suggest, deviance from those norms may have more pronounced consequences among the women.

Do elderly men and women perceive differences in their degree of religiousness? I am not aware of any studies that have looked at this, but some interesting evidence can be found in Kalish and Reynolds (1976). They found, to their surprise, no sex differences in response to their religiosity question, "Compared to most [Anglos, Mexicans, Blacks, Japanese], do you feel you are more, about the same, or less devout?", indicating perhaps that men and women accounted for sex differences before answering.

But differences in the moral content of men's and women's attribution processes are beginning to be noted, and some of the consequences of these differences speculated on. Deaux's (1976) review of studies containing sex as a parameter in the attribution process finds that men and women show differences in attributions for their own behavior and that these differences stem from expectancies based on sex-role stereotypes. Kelley (1971), in fact, explicitly assumes sex-role differences to then look for differences in men's and women's moral evaluations. His classification of causal attributions by their moral basis was discussed in Chapter I. The most interesting part of his argument, however, is its foreshadowing of Carol Gilligan's recently acclaimed *In a Different Voice* (1982). Kelley, an early attribution theorist, outlines three types of moral evaluation: reality-oriented systems (by which he means norms more than moral standards); achievement-oriented systems (geared to mastery over evil forces); and reciprocity-oriented systems (where people consider the effects of their actions on others). The latter two, achievement- and reciprocity-orientation correspond closely to Gilligan's key distinction between an ethic of justice and an ethic of care. She contends that men tend to base their moral decisions on a consideration of the rights of individuals, emphasizing equality, fairness, and justice, while women focus on responsibilities, the relationships between people, and the consequences of their decisions.

These studies, and the fact of women's greater involvement in religion, suggest that men and women may differ in other characteristic attributions as well, in particular the attributions of fatalism and meaning. There is some evidence for this, in McCready and Greeley's (1976) report of NORC data findings that women were both more religious than men, and more likely to be religiously hopeful, while men were most likely to pessimistic or secularly optimistic. One may expect the normatively religious elderly woman even more likely to be religiously hopeful.

Consideration of these sex differences forces consideration of the causes of the differences, a discussion of which cannot even be begun here. The question, to what extent gender relations are based on presumably malleable socialization processes, and to what extent they embody essences that stand outside the social process, will not soon be answered (Rosaldo, 1980). But if men and women make characteristically different attributions for their own and others' motives, for the causes of events and their overall meaning, this could lead the nature/nurture debate into a new phase, by asking, under what circumstances do men and women make characteristically different attributions? In fact researchers have found differences in the attributions women made for the cause of their divorces (it was his fault vs. it was ours) (Langer, 1983), and that men are more analytical and evaluative of their women partners' behavior than women are of men's (Orvis, Kelley, and Butler, 1976). Further clarification of sex differences in attribution processes in descriptive studies such as these will make more precise theoretical explanations possible.

However, some theoretical predictions can be made, based on the functions of religion outlined in this chapter. If an important function of religion for the elderly is to provide meaning for suffering, then one would expect heightened religiosity in identifiable situations of suffering, in poverty, illness, disability, bereavement. Is it possible that women suffer more in old age than men, and hence are more likely to seek comfort in religion?

A basic difference between the sexes is that women live longer than men, seven years on average. Male death rates exceed female death rates at every age from birth, resulting in an over-65 population that has almost one-and-a-half times as many women as men. In the over-80 population, there are almost twice as many women as men (American Public Health Association, 1982, Table 22; U.S.Statistical Abstract, 1979, Table 34). In addition to this, the relative risk of mortality for widowers following bereavement increases sharply (Parkes, Benjamin, and Fitzgerald, 1969), while that for widows remains approximately the same as for married women (Helsing, Szklo, and Comstock, 1981). As a result only 36.7 percent of women over 65 are married and living with their spouse, while more than twice as many men, 74.8 percent, are so situated.

As a recent discussion of the welfare of the American aged has noted, it is women, and especially widows, who predominate among the poorest aged (Crystal, 1982). In 1978, the mean income for men ages 65-69 was $9357; for women it was less than half, $4321 (U.S.Statistical Abstract 1979, Table 754). Social security income drops when a working spouse dies, and some pensions may cease altogether, penalizing elderly widows far more than widowers (Schulz, 1980).

Elderly women are also poorer in health. Despite their favorable mortality risks compared with men, women report higher levels of both mental and physical illness, and utilize health services more often (Nathanson, 1975). In the U.S.Health Interview Survey, women report more bed disability days per year than men do (7.8 compared to 5.6), and more restricted activity days (21.1 compared to 16.9) (American Public Health Association, 1982, Tables 34, 37). They are also less likely than men to describe their health as excellent

(APHA, 1982, Table 31). As admittedly subjective as these measures are, it is impossible to tell whether or not men actually do have better health, or are responding to cultural expectations of stoicism.

A similar, but better studied ambiguity exists regarding women's higher levels of psychological distress in epidemiological surveys. A "sex-role-frustration" hypothesis has been the chief explanation advanced for the nearly universal finding that women are more likely to report being depressed (Gove and Tudor, 1973; Dohrenwend and Dohrenwend, 1976; Gove and Tudor, 1977; Dohrenwend and Dohrenwend, 1977). The thesis has not been easily demonstrated, however (Radloff, 1975; Kessler and McRae, 1981). This issue will be returned to in a later chapter. Here it is enough to suggest that depression be considered, not as a cause of suffering but an indication of it.

This is in fact precisely the rationale for life events research, that depression is a response to exogenous aversive events in life. And women apparently do suffer more of these events than men do; in particular, the loss of a spouse (always considered the most serious life event) and chronic physical illness. In fact women suffer more life events of every kind (Masuda and Holmes, 1978).

A more promising theoretical approach for understanding women's higher levels of psychiatric distress may be the more clinical learned helplessness model of depression (Radloff, 1975) with its attribution theory reformulation. Abramson, Seligman, and Teasdale (1978) and Wheaton (1980) suggest that sex-role-specific attributional styles acquired through socialization may predispose men and women differently to becoming helpless. There is certainly some evidence that men and women respond to life events differently, psychologically and socially. Westbrook and Viney (1983) found women to react to their own serious illness with more anxiety than men, but also with more deliberate socializing. And elderly women were by far the most likely group to respond to their own illness by expressing social solidarity with others.

Two conclusions should be drawn from this recital of the troubles of elderly women. The first is methodological. The situations of men and women with respect to all of the major variables in this study, religious involvement, health, social networks, and attributions of fatalism and meaning, are likely to be so different that all analyses should be carried out separately by sex. Similarity between the two sexes would be the surprising finding.

The second conclusion is the theoretical one, that because women suffer more of life's adverse events, they may be more likely than men to seek religious comfort in theodicies of personal suffering. Wuthnow, Christiano, and Kuzlowski (1980), take a similar position, in hypothesizing that "Personal or intimate imagery of God will be more common among widows than among widowers." The argument here simply is that private religious involvement is particularly relevant in illness, and that women will be more likely than men both to be religious and to be ill. In other words, religion may be more salient for women's health.

This completes a sketch of the ways in which religious theodicies of illness particularize the relationship of religion and health. Because of religion's status as a master sentiment, an overarching structure of belief, it renders the broad range of human misfortune interpretable. There is no human experience which cannot be given religious meaning, for which religion is not a possible way through, not even the experience of dying. This quality of religious involvement should then be most called on by those facing the most misfortune: the bereaved, the ill, and the disabled.

The theodicy hypothesis is thus the fourth and final explanatory hypothesis of the study. In contrast to the three presented in the previous chapter, the health behavior, cohesiveness, and coherence hypotheses, the theodicy hypothesis specifies certain population subgroups for which religious involvement may be expected to be a particularly important psychosocial factor in health. In the first chapter religiosity is predicted to be positively related to all measures of health utilized in the study. This is the argument for the main effect. The hypotheses that there might be a relationship between religion and health because the religiously-involved have better health activities, or larger or more intimate social relations, or a more coherent view of life, are plausible mechanisms by which this association could occur. To the extent that they reduce the association between religion and the measures of health they are evidence of an indirect effect of religious involvement in health, through some other activity or attitude. They help explain the relationship, although they do not explain it away. This analysis could be very helpful in evaluating the relative importance of the psychological and social elements of religion as a psychosocial factor in health. The fourth hypothesis will contribute a test of the idea that psychosocial factors act primarily in interaction with life situations, by providing resources in crises, specifying the test by limiting the situation of stress to that of physical illness, and examining the relationship between religion and psychological distress in conditions of physical illness. Altogether these explanations represent a multidimensional approach to the question of whether and in what ways religious involvement is a significant factor in the health and well-being of the elderly.

III
The Yale Health and Aging Project: Study Design, Measurement, and Analytic Techniques

The Yale Health and Aging Project

The empirical test of the ideas in Chapters I and II will be made with data collected for the Yale Health and Aging Project. Begun in 1980, the Health and Aging Project is a prospective cohort study of 2811 New Haven residents age 65 and over. The broad goals of the Yale Health and Aging Project are to measure the physical health and well-being of the New Haven elderly, and to examine the impact that the social environment has on their health and longevity. To this end, respondents were questioned closely about a broad range of social relationships and interactions, about their families, friends, neighbors, and relatives, and about the frequency, content, and quality of their contacts. The measures of religious involvement thus tap a small subset of the totality of the psychosocial factors in the lives of the elderly. But they are also a microcosm within the big picture; they contain the potential for illustrating all the relevant levels of theoretical explanation of the effect that psychosocial factors may have in health.

The design of the Health and Aging study speaks directly to the methodological issue raised earlier as the biggest obstacle to a clear demonstration of the effects of the social environment on health status. A prospective cohort study, in which health status and social networks alike are measured thoroughly at the baseline, is the single best way to disentangle the effects of health status from social networks. Controlling for health status at the beginning of follow-up, however, is not as straightforward as it may at first appear. In the broad range of measurable mental and physical conditions, there are considerable differences in risk of mortality, and the implications for social network curtailment remain purely speculative. Indeed, some illnesses may not truncate social networks at all; networks can be expanded by mutual aid groups formed by victims of chronic illnesses and their families (Katz and Bender, 1976) or the informal lay referral services for those seeking medical care (Freidson, 1975). A thorough analysis of adequate measures of both health and social networks at baseline, combined with careful follow-up of the cohort, offer the surest methodological foundation for inferring the effects of social networks on the health of individuals.

The overall goal in selecting the cohort to be studied was to fairly represent the population of elderly people who live independently in the community, that is, in non-institutionalized settings. A stratified sample was drawn from the three predominant types of housing in which the elderly live: from private homes interspersed throughout the community, from public elderly housing where residents are both age- and income-restricted, and from privately-sponsored elderly housing whose residents are restricted by age only. As can be seen in Table III-1., the three groups in the sample are somewhat alike in average age and education, but quite different in other demographic characteristics. The respondents living in public housing are mostly women, unmarried, with low incomes, and almost half are nonwhite. The private elderly housing sample is nearly all white; again women outnumber the men and most of these women are unmarried. The non-age-segregated housing sample has the highest average income levels and proportion of married respondents. The qualitative differences between the three strata make controlling for this sampling design variable mandatory in all multivariate analyses.

The remainder of this chapter is a description of the measures used in the interviews, the indices specially constructed for the analyses, and an overall view of the analytic strategy employed.

Table III-1. Demographic characteristics of the
Yale Health and Aging Project sample
New Haven, Connecticut, 1982

Characteristic	Age (mean years)	Race (% white)	Income (% < $5000)	Education (mean years)	Marital Status (% married)	TOTAL N
PUBLIC HOUSING						
Men	74.6	54.8	47.9	10.4	32.3	239
Women	75.6	54.0	64.9	10.3	15.4	489
PRIVATE HOUSING						
Men	74.9	95.2	21.3	10.1	52.3	331
Women	75.3	90.3	40.6	11.2	17.0	537
OTHER HOUSING						
Men	73.1	84.7	14.2	10.2	71.9	596
Women	74.1	83.0	29.8	10.7	33.4	619
TOTAL	74.5	78.8	35.1	10.4	37.5	2811

The Religion and Health Subset of the Data

The subset of the data that will be used in the following analyses includes only the completed interviews; no interviews which the respondent was unable to complete, or interviews in which a proxy gave the responses are included. Thus 55 respondents of the total 2811 are excluded, yielding a total N for the subset of 2756. Because the religion variables are central to the analysis, those respondents who failed to answer these questions are, in effect, also excluded. There were 35 such individuals, 11 men and 24 women, making up just 1.3% of the sample. They tended to be older and in poorer health, which is not surprising considering that the questions come near the end of a fairly lengthy interview. A more important limitation, however, is that the data set includes only the responses to the baseline questionnaire.

Thus the study design for the present analysis of religion and health is cross-sectional, a level of analysis appropriate for the highly exploratory nature of the hypotheses. A thorough analysis at the baseline is a mandatory prerequisite for further longitudinal analyses. The following variables and indices are those chosen for analysis.

Health Status
        There are four variables which measure health status: an index of chronic conditions, an index of functional disability, a scale measuring depressive feelings, and a direct query about the respondent's perception of his or her own health. The measures were carefully selected to span the objective-subjective dimension of health status, and to build on each other, as the objective measures have some bearing on subjective perceptions. So, for example, the number of chronic conditions an individual reports will be used as a control in the analysis of functional disability, and chronic conditions and functional disability will act as controls in the analysis of depression, and so on.

Chronic Conditions Index. This index is a simple, unweighted sum of positive responses to questions about the major chronic illnesses of the elderly. The eleven conditions include myocardial infarction, cerebral hemorrhage, cancer, diabetes, cirrhosis, fractured hip, other broken bones (indicating osteoporosis), hypertension, arthritis, Parkinson's Disease, and amputation of a limb. Respondents scored "1" if they reported a doctor's diagnosis of the condition, "0" if they did not; the small number of non-diagnosed but suspected cases were also given a "1." The "1"s were then summed over the conditions, resulting in possible scores that range from 0 to 11. If the respondent failed to answer an individual item they were scored as not having the condition. None of the respondents in the subset failed to answer all items, so all received a score on the index. This is the most objective of the health measures in that it requires the least amount of judgment on the respondent's part. It is unweighted to reflect the tension between those conditions for which the risk of mortality is high, and those for which the risk of mortality is low but the risk of disability is high.

Functional Disability Index. The measure of disability used in the present study was adapted directly from several scales used in earlier studies of both the general population, and the elderly specifically.

Seven activities of daily living (ADL), designed to assess the ability of the elderly to live independently, were adapted from Katz, Downs, Cash, and Grotz (1970). These include the ability of the respondent to walk across a small room, to bathe, groom, dress, eat, get from bed to a chair, and use the toilet, without help or much difficulty. Three gross mobility activities were included, doing heavy work around the house, getting up and down stairs, and walking half a mile, (Rosow and Breslau, 1966), as were five physical activities from the work of Nagi (1976): the ability to move large furniture, to stoop or kneel, carry weights of ten pounds or less, reach above shoulder level, and write or handle small objects. These fifteen activities approximately correspond to those which were the subject of the Framingham Disability Study (Jette and Branch, 1981).

There are substantial differences between deficits in the first group, which are self-care activities minimally required for independent living, and in the latter two, which are more optional measures of agility and endurance. For this reason, three separate scales were originally constructed, one for the most basic activities of daily living (Katz), the second for mobility (Rosow), and the third for the more minor physical activities (Nagi).

For the first, respondents were considered unable to do the activity if they required help from another person or special equipment. Respondents who currently required help in, or were completely unable to do any one of the seven self-care activities scored a "1" for the subscale as a whole, because it was felt that the activities like eating, bathing, and moving across a room were so basic that an indication of having any trouble at all was significant. If the respondent could perform all activities without help they scored "0."

The second scale is made up of three Rosow-Breslau (1966) gross mobility items. No fine distinctions were made for doing heavy housework, climbing a flight of steps or walking half a mile; respondents either were or were not able to. If respondents were unable to do one of the activities, they scored "1" for the subscale.

For the five physical activity items (Nagi, 1976), respondents who reported any difficulty were grouped with those having great difficulty or unable to do the activity at all. Thus respondents reporting difficulty in moving furniture, kneeling, lifting, raising their arms, or handling small objects received a "1" on the subscale. For each of the three subscales, if respondents were missing all items, they were considered missing on the subscale.

A summary index of functional disability was created by combining these three scales, capitalizing on their powers of discrimination across a wide range of physical activities from the most minimally necessary to some which would be moderately strenuous. At one end of the scale are grouped all those who needed any help in even one of the Katz Activities of Daily Living. At the other end are those who had no difficulty with any of the Katz, Rosow, or Nagi physical activity items. The five-level summary index was created in the following way: if an individual scored "0" on all subscales, they were considered free of disability and scored "1" on the index. If they scored "1" on the Nagi subscale, but "0" on the Rosow and Katz subscales, they scored "2". If they scored "1" on the Rosow subscale, but "0" on the Nagi and Katz subscales they scored "3." If they scored "1" on both the Nagi and Rosow subscales, they scored "4." And if they scored "1" on all three subscales, indicating the highest level of disability, they received a "5" on the summary disability index. Seventy-four respondents were missing.

Depression Symptoms Scale. The measurement of depressive feelings is the widely-used Center for Epidemiologic Studies Depression Scale. The 20-item scale is reproduced in Appendix A. Responses to each item are scored from "1" to "4" depending on how often the respondent felt that way in the previous week, and the final score is an unweighted sum of all responses. Respondents who failed to answer one or two of the items were included by prorating the missing items with the average of the 19 or 18 answered items. Respondents failing to answer three or more items were considered missing. Scores could thus range from 20 (low) to 80 (high). Seventy-nine respondents were missing.

Self-Assessment of Health. This measure of health status is simply the answer to the question "How would you rate your health at the present time?" The coded choices are: 1) Excellent, 2) Good, 3) Fair, 4) Poor, and 5) Bad. As such it is the most subjective measure of health, tapping a more generalized state of well-being than do the objective measures of physical health. Twenty-four respondents were missing.

Religious Involvement
        There are five questions pertaining to religion in the questionnaire. The items are analyzed individually, and in addition,

two indices are created, one measuring public religious involvement and one measuring private religious involvement.

1. What is your religious preference? 1) Catholic 2) Protestant
   3) Jewish 4) Other 5) None

The first religion variable is religious preference. Recent research in the sociology of religion is very consistent in finding that, among Catholics, Protestants, Jews, and others, there is more within-group variation on many major political and social issues than there is between groups (Herberg, 1960). Evidence of mental health differences between groups has already been presented. There may also be a difference between individuals who profess any religious group identification at all, and those who profess none. The operative distinction may be that of having any religious group affiliation, no matter how unexercised. At the very least such an identification indicates that the individual recognizes potential communities of fellow believers to which he or she could turn.

2. About how often do you go to religious meetings or services?
   1) Never/almost never 2) Once or twice a year 3) Every few months 4) Once or twice a month 5) Once a week 6) More than once a week

This variable is minimally the indication of potential for meeting people and having some social interaction, if not an indication of interaction itself. It also indicates participation in the public devotional and ritual acts of the religious body, an expression of solidarity with the religious community. Attending religious services gives one a period during which the self is partially lost in the group as a whole, when reflection on one's life and relationships is encouraged, and thanks may be given or resolution for problems sought. It is thus the most important measure of both the integration and the regulation of the cohesiveness hypothesis.

3. How many people in your congregation do you know personally?
   1) None 2) A few 3) Many 4) Almost all

This question, theoretically a measure of social involvement with the religious group, may be to a large extent more a reflection of church or temple congregation size than an indication of the individual respondent's sociability. The smaller the group, the more likely an individual is to know a high proportion of other members. Nevertheless, religious service attendance and social connections with other congregation members are the available measures of the social cohesiveness of religion for the elderly of New Haven. These are the social structures that vitiate the egoism and anomie: the formal, ritualized intercourse with the religious body as a whole, and the informal, not necessarily religiously-based interactions within that structure.

4. Aside from attendance at religious services, do you consider yourself to be... 1) Deeply religious 2) Fairly religious 3) Only slightly religious 4) Not at all religious 5) Against religion

This is the question of religious identity, how does one think of oneself. The answer "I am deeply religious" reveals a certain amount of reflection, introspection, and self-awareness. On the other hand, it is an identification that was public and socially acceptable enough to the respondent that he or she openly admitted it. For the elderly, whose social roles are diminishing in number, the religious identity may become increasingly important. Beyond the self-perception of identity, both this question and the next may be seen as indications of an experiential element of religion, as well as a feeling of belonging.

5. How much is religion a source of strength and comfort to you? 1) None 2) A little 3) A great deal

While the previous question alludes to the depth or intensity of religious experience, this one asks whether or not such experience has a positive effect. Receiving strength and comfort from religion is likely to be associated with times in which such comfort would be sought, that is, in periods of suffering. Acknowledgement of such solace may also indicate a certain amount of religious certainty, or salvation, which for Weber (1922) is closely linked to the concept of theodicy.

Public Religiosity Index. To facilitate a test of the social cohesiveness hypothesis, religion items 2 and 3 were combined into a single measure. The responses for each item were first divided by the highest score possible for the item, and then summed, resulting in a scale with a possible high score of "2." Respondents failing to answer one question received a zero for that question; those failing to answer both were considered missing.

Private Religiosity Index. To facilitate a test of the coherence hypothesis, a similar index was created from religion items 4 and 5. It was necessary to reverse the codings for the question about religious identity, and the very few responding that they were "against religion" were combined with those saying they were "not at all religious." The responses were again weighted and summed, resulting in a possible high score of "2."

Health Practices
        The following four measures are indications of health habits or a healthy lifestyle, and as such comprise the test of the health behavior hypothesis. They are all treated separately in the analyses.

Quetelet Index. This is intended as a measure of overweight. Weight (in pounds) is standardized by height (in inches), squared.

Alcohol Consumption Index. This is a measure of the volume of beer, wine, and liquor the respondent consumed during the previous month. Each type of drink (beer, wine, liquor) is weighted by the average number of drinks the respondent had at one time, and the number of times during the previous month that the respondent drank. The weighted components are then summed.

Physical Activity Index. This is a combined measure of the frequency with which the respondent swims or engages in active sports, takes walks, works in the garden, or does physical exercise. Responses are coded 1) often, 2) sometimes, and 3) never. Codings were reversed to make the higher scores indicate more activity, and sports/swimming, taking walks, and exercising were given twice the weight (2, 4, or 6) of working in the garden. Responses were then summed.

Smoking. Respondents were simply classified into three groups: present smokers, those who had quit, and those who had never smoked.

Social Networks
    The set of measures used to test the social cohesiveness hypothesis were in general chosen to represent generic structural features of social networks rather than specific types of relationships.

Size Index. This is the most encompassing social network indicator, a simple counting-up of all the major relationships an individual names as people they feel close to. It includes the spouse, children, relatives, close friends and neighbors. Each tie is weighted equally and scores "1," so that for example, a married woman with three children, a sister, a brother, and nine close friends or neighbors would score "15" on the size index.

Contact Index. This measure is somewhat more restrictive, limiting network ties to those where regular contacts are actually made. It includes the number of their children that the individual sees, talks to on the phone, or corresponds with at least once a week; the number of relatives the individual sees or corresponds with at least several times a year; and the number of friends the individual sees at least once a month, or corresponds with several times a year. Again, all ties are weighted equally, so that if the woman in the previous example lived with her husband, saw all of her children, friends, and neighbors frequently, but did not correspond with her brother or sister, she would score "13" on the contact index.

Friends Index. This is the number of non-kin ties, the total of close friends and neighbors the individual knows well enough to visit in their homes. The same woman would score "9" here.

Intimacy Index. This is a very restrictive measure. Only an individual's closest and most intimate relationships are counted here, their confidant and those of their children that they feel *very* close to. If the woman considered her husband her confidant, and felt very close to all of her children, her intimacy score would be "4."

Marital Status. Finally there is marital status, an important demographic category, as well as a social network indicator. For the analyses, respondents were classified in one of three groups: presently married, formerly married, or never married.

Sense of Coherence

The test of the coherence hypothesis is made with two indices created from six attitude items in the questionnaire. The original six items were these:

1. Many things that have happened to me are the result of luck.
2. Even though I don't always understand why things happen, I have faith that they will turn out all right.
3. When I look back I feel my life has had no plan or order to it.
4. I have always had a sense that I belong, that I was a part of things.
5. I think this world is out of control.
6. I feel completely helpless.
   Rarely or none of the time - 1
   Some of the time - 2
   Much of the time - 3
   Most or all of the time - 4

The correlation matrix and subsequent factor analysis of these items identified two factors, one made up of items 2 and 4, the other made up of items 1, 3, and 6. Item 5 was not highly correlated with the other items.

Meaning Index. This measure is the sum of the responses to items 2 and 4. If an individual missed one item, they received the score for the item they answered. If they missed both items, they were considered missing. The higher the score, the greater the sense of meaning. These items contain the ideas of a confidence and hope in the future, even in the midst of a present which may be troubling or difficult to understand. The other element is a feeling of belonging, a sense of being one among others, a part of something larger than oneself. The high correlation of these two items (Pearson $r = .40$) is an interesting finding in itself. Together, they correspond well with the definition of the attribution of meaning developed earlier. Without indicating a schema of values, beliefs, or symbols, they imply that the individual possesses some cognitive resource for coping with the present that allows for a sense of ultimate, if not immediate, resolution. And they indicate a view of the world that is seen as shared by others.

Fatalism Index. To create this index, the codings for items 1, 3, and 6 were reversed so that when summed, the lower scores represent the greater sense of fatalism. Again, individuals missing one or two items were included; individuals missing three were considered missing. This measure is comprised of the idea of a lack of the individual's control over events without any suggestion that that control is centered anywhere else; a sense that one's life has been muddled through, rather than conceived and executed; and an unambiguous sense of helplessness. Though not as high as the correlation of the items in the Meaning Index, the correlations among these items (Pearson r=(1-3):.25 (1-6):.27 (3-6):.30) and their identification as a factor support the integrity of the fatalism construct.

Table III-2. presents the univariate statistics for the major variables in the study.

Analytic Strategies

The major goals of the analysis are these: 1) to describe the patterns of religious participation of the New Haven elderly; 2) to describe the associations between the various forms of religious participation and a)health practices, b)social networks, and c)attributions of meaning and fatalism; 3) to describe the associations between the various forms of religious participation and the various measures of health; and 4) to test the health behavior, cohesion, coherence, and theodicy hypotheses as intervening factors in those relationships.

The first step in the analysis was a preliminary survey of the bivariate relationships of each religion variable with all other variables in the data set. At this stage, continuous measurements were treated as interval data. Crosstabulation tables were carefully examined for general trends, as well as the contribution of individual cells to the chi square statistics.

Table III-2. Health, religion, health practice, social network
and coherence characteristics of the health and religion
subset of the Yale Health and Aging Project data

Variable	Value Range	Mean	S.D.
HEALTH STATUS			
Chronic conditions	0-7 Conditions	1.74	1.24
Functional disability	1 (disability) - 5 (severe disability)	2.62	1.48
Depression	20 (no depression) - 77	28.35	8.51
Self-assessed health	1 (excellent) - 5 (bad)	2.39	0.84
RELIGION			
Religious preference	53% Catholic, 29% Protestant, 14% Jewish, 3% Other, 1% None		
Attendance	1 (Never attends) - 6 (more than once a week)	3.36	1.74
Knows congregation	1 (knows no one) - 4 (knows everyone)	2.45	0.98
Religious identity	1 (deeply religious) - 5 (against religion)	1.81	0.78
Religious comfort	1 (no comfort) - 3 (a great deal)	2.64	0.60
Public religiosity	0 (least) - 2 (most)	1.19	0.47
Private religiosity	0 (least) - 2 (most)	1.67	0.36
HEALTH BEHAVIORS			
Quetelet index	1.0 (light) - 29.9 (heavy)	5.77	2.29
Alcohol use index	0.0 (doesn't drink) - 180	10.56	18.28
Activity index	0.0 (most inactive) - 14 (most active)	4.00	3.03
Smoking status	20% present smokers, 29% past smokers, 50% never smoked		
SOCIAL NETWORKS			
Size index	0.0 (no one) - 99 *	11.15	9.40
Contact index	0.0 (no one) - 99 *	12.28	10.99
Friends index	0.0 (no one) - 99 *	6.02	7.36
Intimacy index	0.0 (no one) - 15	2.55	1.90
Marital status	37% married, 4% separated, 7% divorced, 42% widowed, 10% never		
COHERENCE			
Meaning index	1 (least meaning) - 8 (most)	6.37	1.95
Fatalism index	1 (most fatalistic) - 12 (least)	9.53	2.30

* values greater than 99 reduced to 99

The second step was a thorough analysis of the independent variables. Using first general linear regression/correlation models and then log linear models, the relationships of the various types of religious involvement to the separate components of the study's hypotheses were analyzed. The regression models were derived using the SAS General Linear Models program, (1982 Edition), the log linear models with BMDP4F. The advantages of the first method nicely complement those of the second. Multiple regression/correlation can handle a large number of variables, and models may contain both continuous and categorical variables. Moreover, SAS GLM will generate parameter estimates for each level of specified class variables, and even allow continuous or class variables to be nested within class variables, permitting detailed examination of significant interactions.

The substantive difference between the multiple regression/correlation models and the log linear models is that the former necessarily impose a structure of factors and response on the variables, whereas the log linear models assess all the possible statistical associations between all the variables simultaneously. There are no responses or factors; each variable is potentially of equal importance. Developed as a way of dealing with categorical variables, the log linear technique (BMDP4F) is thus especially appropriate for the exploratory analysis of cross-sectional data sets. The disadvantage of the technique is that there are limits on the number of variables that can be included in a model, and also on the number of levels those variables can take on. Thus the results of the more comprehensive multiple regression/correlation models were weighed carefully in choosing the variables for the log linear analysis. The two approaches differ in that one makes broad sweeps through the data and the other makes a more penetrating foray into a cluster of variables that is of particular interest.

The third and final step was to derive multiple regression/correlation models for each of the measures of health status, assessing the significance of their relationship with the religion variables and testing the behavioral, social cohesiveness, sense of coherence, and theodicy hypotheses as mediators of the association. The general procedure followed in model-construction was a hierarchical analysis using sets of variables (Cohen and Cohen, 1983). The first model contains the set of religion variables, the indices of public and private religiosity (housing stratum having been entered first as a blocking factor in consideration of the sampling design). The second model introduces the demographic factors. The third model adds the health behavior measures, introducing all the health practice variables while retaining significant demographic factors and the two religiosity indices. The fourth model enters the social cohesiveness variables examining changes in the religiosity indices when the social network variables are introduced and the previously significant health behavior and demographic factors retained. Fifth, the sense of coherence measures are added, introducing the meaning and fatalism terms and examining changes in the religiosity indices. The sixth model adds the relevant health status controls which build on each other in the cumulative manner described earlier; the more objective health status measures become part of the models for the more subjective health measures. Finally, the theodicy hypothesis is tested with interactions of the individual religion variables and the health status measures.

Strictly speaking, hierarchical analysis usually orders variables or variable sets by causal priority; that is, no variable entering at a later step should be considered a presumptive cause of an earlier variable (Cohen and Cohen, 1983). Followed precisely, such a sequencing would begin with the most stable background factors, proceed to the focal variables of the study, and finish with any exploratory hypotheses. Such a strategy maximizes the usefulness of the model R^2 and partial correlation statistics. The information yielded by the progression of models is vastly richer than that which would be obtained by entering all variables simultaneously.

The order of variable set entry for the present study described above, however, while capitalizing on the logic of hierarchical analysis, openly violates its rule by introducing the health controls at the last step rather than at the first or second. This modification was intentional, though, and requires an explanation. The crucial importance of controlling for health level in the analysis of social factors in health has been repeatedly emphasized. And with respect to the final model, it makes no difference whether health status was controlled from the beginning or added at the last step. It is the intermediate results that are affected. Bearing in mind, then, the tenuousness of the intermediate steps, it was still felt that the analysis would be more instructive if the results could be viewed both with and without the health controls. In this way one could see what might have been. Potential errors in interpretation will be revealed and acknowledged rather than being prevented and remaining mysterious. Moreover, it can be assumed that the health controls will add considerable variance to the models when introduced, and it would be an advantage to compare partial and semipartial correlation coefficients, and total model R^2s before and after introduction of the health controls.

The order of introduction of the health behavior, social cohesiveness, and coherence variable sets does follow the hierarchical analysis rule. The risks associated with the health behaviors are by far the best known and most reliably measured. And while they cannot be considered proximate causes of the other two hypotheses, most would agree that their effects should be taken into account first, making the tests of the cohesiveness, coherence, and theodicy hypotheses more stringent.

If any associations between religion and health are found, interpretation must be cautious. Because this is a cross-sectional data set, the language of regression analysis, with its factor and response terms, could easily imply causal direction when in fact none can be established. It would be incorrect to speak of these models "predicting health outcomes," or showing the "effects of psychosocial factors on health" when both psychosocial factors and health status were measured simultaneously. Even the more neutral terms "independent" and "dependent" variable indicate a sort of causal hierarchy, although they also suggest, correctly, that the analyst has set up the problem by deciding which shall be which. Hence, interpretation of these models must be circumspect, and while conventional criteria for causal order, i.e. time order, plausible intervening mechanisms, monotonic trends, etc., will be discussed, no premature conclusions about the ultimate relationship of religion and health will be reached.

The major contribution of the analysis, in any case, will not be the results of these individual models, but the comparisons which will be made between and among them. The two indices of religion used here, and their components, are substantively different from each other and have not been used in epidemiological studies before. The way they will act with each other, with the health measures, and with the different demographic groups is unknown and must be carefully described before more conclusive longitudinal studies can be undertaken. The virtue of cross-sectional studies is that they are descriptive. They plot out relationships on a conceptual map that can only be two-dimensional. No hierarchy can be legitimately imposed on these relationships when all points are plotted at the same time, but to impose the methodological hierarchy of a longitudinal study on variables whose relationships at a stable point in time are not well understood would be to ride roughshod over what may be subtle but important phenomena. The most responsible interpretation of these analyses will be one that is extremely conservative and highly detailed.

The results of the analysis will be reported in the next five chapters. Chapter IV presents the results of the analyses of the independent variables, and the analyses of the health measures begin in Chapter V.

IV
The Conditions of
Religious Participation

The relationship of the independent variables to each other is an issue often raised only at the end of a sociological analysis, as a check on the validity of the findings. When the study population is a sample of an entire community, however, this cheats the analysis of color and concreteness. It also increases the likelihood of making misleading interpretations of the data. The purpose of this chapter is to develop the shades of meaning of the forms of involvement in religion by describing what they are associated with, that is, whether sex and age, for example, really do make a difference in religious involvement, as the literature leads one to expect. The patterns of religious involvement of men and women will be compared, as will those of the major ethnic-religious groups in New Haven. The comparisons will be made with frequency tables and chi square statistics weighted by 1980 census tract figures to compensate for oversampling in particular areas, and thus may be considered representative of the population of New Haven as a whole. Second, the relationship of men's and women's religious involvement to their health behaviors, social networks, and senses of coherence will be analyzed in analysis of variance tables (with unweighted data). Finally, log linear analyses of men's and women's religious involvement, social networks, and senses of coherence are performed and the patterns for the two sexes compared. In this way a foundation can be laid for the analyses of health measures that follow.

Age and Sex Differences in Religion

Knowledge of the religious involvement patterns of the elderly has been limited, more than anything else, by small numbers that force researchers to group all those over 65 into one or two categories. Yet any empirical assessment of Bahr's (1970) four models of aging and religious disaffiliation requires substantial numbers of the elderly in

77

their sixties, seventies, eighties, and nineties. The best evidence is that there is some decline in public religious participation with age; but is it a slow, steady decline from age 65 on, or is there a period of stability that continues the patterns of middle age before a decline begins? And does private religious involvement remain stable, or increase in some relationship to the decline in public involvement? Figure IV-1. presents the age curves for the major religious groups, showing the large number of respondents in the sample who are well into their eighties and nineties, and the relative sizes of the major religious groups, Catholics, Protestants, Jews, and others. "Other" includes Greek, Russian and Ukrainian Orthodox, and independent churches. Only above age 90 do the numbers of respondents get very small. Figure IV-1. and all the following figures are weighted by 1980 census tract data to compensate for oversampling in particular areas, and thus do represent the population of New Haven as a whole.

Figure IV-2. shows the proportion of each five-year age group that attends religious services at least once a week. As one would expect, there are more women attending regularly than men in every age group but one, and substantially more at the youngest ages. Although the men and the women do display a modified stability-decline pattern, the highest proportion of regular attenders among both the men and the women comes not in the youngest age group, but among those 70-74. A sharp decline in regular attendance occurs for both sexes in the 90+ age group; before that, there are apparently random fluctuations. This is not evidence of an age effect--no such interpretation can be made with cross-sectional data such as these. But if the data are consistent with the stability-decline model, the very late age of the beginning of the decline in attendance is notable. Moreover, the rather high proportions of regular attenders, (35-40 percent), among the near-centenarians casts doubt on the presumed inevitability of the decline. Thus the only evidence for an age effect in reducing attendance at religious services is modest, and the decline is evident only at the oldest ages.

Figure IV-3. shows less decline in religious involvement when the indicator used is the number of people the respondent knows in their congregation. At most ages, about the same proportion of women and men know most of those in their congregations. At the oldest ages, men tend to know more congregation members than women do. The proportion of women saying they know many of those in their congregation declines after age 74, from 57 percent to 45 percent. The

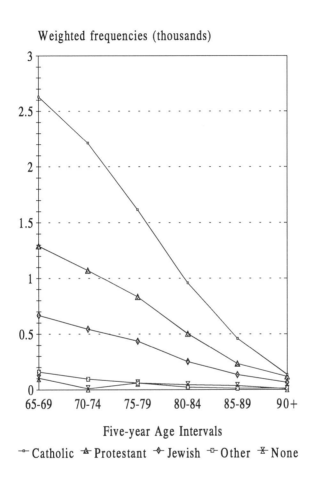

Figure IV-1.
Weighted frequency distribution of age
groups by religious affiliation

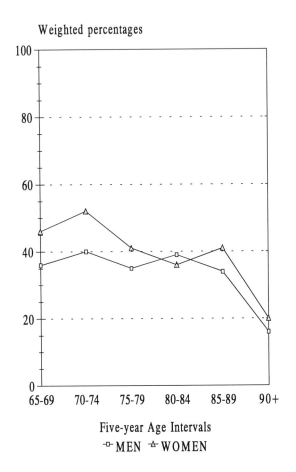

Figure IV-2.
Weighted percentages in 5-year age groups attending
religious services once a week or more often

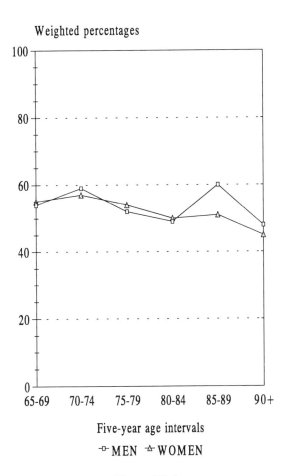

Figure IV-3.
Weighted percentages in 5-year age groups
knowing many or all in their congregation

men's pattern is erratic; the highest proportion of men knowing many comes in the 85-89 year age group.

Figure IV-4. shows the proportion of men and women at each age group who identify themselves as being deeply religious. At every age, more women than men think of themselves as being deeply religious. But even more striking is the similarity between the sexes: with only one exception, there is a steadily increasing proportion of deeply religious people at every older age. In other words, more and more of the people who live to the oldest ages have a deeply religious identity. Again, this cannot be considered an age effect, but the regularity of the increase makes it harder to dismiss out-of-hand as a cohort effect.

The first thing to notice about Figure IV-5. is the very high level of the percentages of respondents who say they receive a great deal of strength and comfort from religion. It says very simply that not only those people who attend religious services regularly and who have an active social involvement in their church or temple receive such strength and comfort from religion. Apparently there are some who receive such solace without such public religious involvement. The proportions also greatly surpass those who say they are deeply religious. Being comforted by religion, then, is the most prevalent form of religious involvement considered here, among both men and women. More women than men feel that they get a great deal of strength and comfort from religion, about 77 percent of every age group. For the men, on the other hand, the proportion rises steadily in the older age groups.

Does religious involvement depend at all on age? The only declining religious involvement here is modest and begins very late. The most significant correlation between age and any of these religion variables, however, is between age and religious identity ($r = .09$, $p < .01$ for both men and women), and that is a positive correlation; religious identity *increases* with age. Thus evidence for a hypothesis of religious disengagement with age is lacking.

Ethnic-Religious Differences

New Haven, Connecticut, where the study was carried out, is a religiously-diverse community whose religious groups tend also to be split along ethnic lines. There are four major ethnic-religious groups in

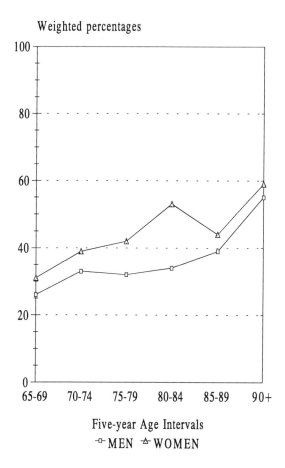

Figure IV-4.
Weighted percentages in 5-year age groups
saying they were deeply religious

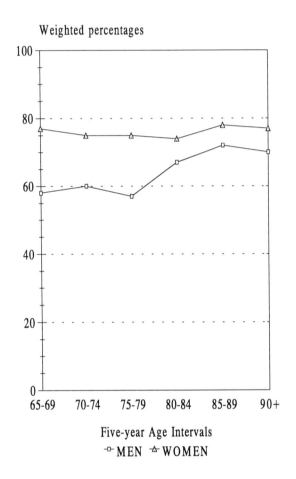

Figure IV-5.
Weighted percentages in 5-year age groups saying they
receive a great deal of strength and comfort from religion

New Haven: white Catholics, the largest group, and about equal numbers of black Protestants, Jews, and white Protestants. This is a peculiarly urban, even Northeastern urban distribution that is very different from the U.S. population as a whole, where 59 percent are Protestant and only 28 percent are Roman Catholic (Princeton Religion Research Center, 1982). These four ethnic-religious groups tend to have distinctly different patterns of religious involvement, thus the importance of their relative weight in this sample must be kept in mind. Again, the figures given in the tables are weighted to correspond with the New Haven population.

Table IV-1. Percentage frequency distribution of religious service attendance of major ethnic-religious groups, weighted

Attendance	White Catholics	Black Protestants	Jews	White Protestants	Total
Never	19.9	13.8	17.7	35.8	20.9%
1-2/Year	9.9	8.9	25.4	14.9	12.8%
3-10/Year	8.2	10.3	30.2	10.9	12.3%
1-2/Month	8.7	22.8	8.4	12.0	11.2%
Once/Week	48.5	32.2	14.6	19.3	36.8%
More than once	4.7	12.0	3.7	7.1	6.0%
Total	100%	100%	100%	100%	100%
Weighted N	7661	2006	2094	1926	13690

It can be seen in Table IV-1. that regular attendance at religious services is significantly greater in some groups than in others $X^2 = 2467.2$, $p < .0001$). White Catholics are typically once-a-week attenders. They are both the largest group (over half the population) and the group with the largest percentage attending once a week or more often (53 percent). Black Protestants, Jews, and white Protestants are approximately equal-sized groups. Black Protestants also have a high level of regular attendance; 44 percent attend once a week or more, 67 percent attend once a month or more. Jews are most likely to attend services every few months, a pattern of observing religious holidays but not regular sabbaths. In contrast to all three, white Protestants are largely non-attenders. Thirty-six percent never attend services at all, and only 26 percent attend once a week or more. Thus the predominant ethnic-religious group is also the most assiduous in its religious practice, and the Roman Catholic norm of attending mass weekly thus pushes up attendance levels in the population as a whole.

Table IV-2. shows the ethnic-religious groups' patterns of knowing the other members of their congregation. These differences are also significant ($X^2 = 1126.3$, p. < .0001). The biggest deviation from the expected pattern comes for the white Protestants, who are disproportionately likely to say they do not know anyone at all in their congregation. Black Protestants, on the other hand, are disproportionately likely to say they know every one. Jews, also, tend to know more people rather than fewer. Surprisingly, the majority group of Catholics, for all their attendance at services, tends to fall on the side of knowing fewer, not more; the expected number say they know many, fewer than expected say they know all. This may be explained in part by the size of congregations, Roman Catholic churches tending to be larger, black Protestant churches smaller and more intimate. But it also underscores the fact that there is no perfect concomitance between attendance at services and social involvement with others in the congregation, though admittedly the correlation between the two is high (r = .54, p < .0001).

Table IV-2. Percentage frequency distribution of number of fellow congregants known by major ethnic-religious groups, weighted

	White Catholics	Black Protestants	Jews	White Protestants	Total
No one	17.2	6.7	12.8	33.8	17.3%
A few	32.3	23.5	17.6	21.7	27.3%
Many	41.9	44.5	55.5	29.4	42.6%
All	8.6	25.2	14.0	15.1	12.8%
Total	100%	100%	100%	100%	100%
Weighted N	7418	1962	2025	1874	13279

In Table IV-3. we see the distribution of feelings of religiousness. Again the differences are highly significant ($X^2 = 1368.4$, p < .0001). This time it is the Jews who deviate most from the expected pattern; many fewer than expected think of themselves as being deeply religious. Jews and white Protestants are both disproportionately likely to say they are not religious at all. It is white Catholics and black Protestants who are most likely to say they are deeply religious.

The correlation of the two private forms of religious involvement, religious identity and receiving strength and comfort from religion, is slightly stronger than that between the public forms, knowing other congregants and attendance, $r = .58$, ($p < .0001$) vs. $r = .54$ ($p < .0001$). The proportion of each ethnic-religious group that feels they receive a great deal of solace from religion is shown in Table IV-4. As can be seen, the very high overall proportion of people feeling that they receive a great deal of strength from religion is not equally distributed through the groups ($X^2 = 1689.8$, $p < .0001$). Both white Catholics and black Protestants are overwhelmingly likely to feel that they get a great deal of comfort, but fewer white Protestants and only 38 percent of Jews say they do. Nevertheless, these are all substantial proportions, and less than 6 percent of the group as a whole say they get no comfort from religion at all.

Table IV-3. Percentage frequency distribution of self-expressed religiousness of major ethnic-religious groups, weighted

	White Catholics	Black Protestants	Jews	White Protestants	Total
Not religious	.9	.1	7.4	6.5	2.7%
Slightly	8.8	4.4	24.0	12.5	11.0%
Fairly	47.1	48.8	55.9	54.1	49.6%
Deeply	43.2	45.9	12.7	26.8	36.7%
Total	100%	100%	100%	100%	100%
Weighted N	7635	1988	2077	1885	13585

On balance, it is black Protestants who emerge as the most religiously-involved. More black Protestants than any other ethnic-religious group attend church at least once a month, know everyone in their congregations, think of themselves as deeply religious, and receive a great deal of strength and comfort from religion. As a substantially large ethnic-religious group in the city, they combine with the Roman Catholics to set very high levels of religiosity in the population as a whole, a possible peculiarity of the data which must be kept in mind.

Table IV-4. Percentage frequency distribution of perceived
strength and comfort from religion of
major ethnic-religious groups, weighted

	White Catholics	Black Protestants	Jews	White Protestants	Total
None	2.9	.5	15.9	10.5	5.6%
A little	19.8	12.2	45.6	27.9	23.7%
A great deal	77.3	87.3	38.5	61.6	70.7%
Total	100%	100%	100%	100%	100%
Weighted N	7561	1998	2030	1893	13482

Religious Involvement and the Health Behaviors

Do the health practices of the more religiously-involved differ
from those of the less involved? As the literature review indicated, very
little is known about this relationship, so the simple description of
findings is of some interest. But one must also approach the issue
substantively and ask if the particular religious groups found in New
Haven hold religious doctrines that could be interpreted as health
practices. In a way, this may seem like an overly fine point, but it gets
at a very basic matter of definition. Asking about the health practices
of religious groups implies that a value is placed on health by the
religious group, an assumption which may be valid in some cases but
should not be assumed for all. A more precise framing of the question
would be, are there religious teachings prescribing or proscribing
religious activities which also function as health practices in reducing
known health risk factors? From the point of view of religious doctrine,
the health advantages of such practices is irrelevant.[1] Religious
practices that are also health practices are thus a specific indication of
moral regulation, and in a sense form a sub-hypothesis that combines
elements of the health behavior hypothesis and the social network
hypothesis. In fact it is this very substantive similarity that permitted
Gardner and Lyon (1982) to so blithely take social location within the
Mormon church as an indicator of adherence to church dietary
practices.

In point of fact, however, none of the major religious
traditions represented in New Haven, with the possible exception of

Orthodox Jews or Baptists, prescribe or proscribe any of the particular health practices in question: smoking, alcohol consumption, overweight, or physical exercise. Thus any associations between religious involvement and these health activities must be explained on grounds other than formal doctrinal teaching. Any interpretation of such an association might be speculatively based on a general Judeo-Christian tradition of respect for human life and the physical body[2], but a convincing argument must await further research.

What, then, are the associations of religious involvement with the health practices in the data? For each of the four health behavior variables, tests of association with the religious involvement variables were made with multiple regression/correlation models. Four separate models were run, one for each of the health behaviors. All independent variables were entered simultaneously. Housing stratum was controlled, sex was included as a dummy variable, and the religion variables were treated as class variables so that parameter estimates for each level could be examined. The results, for each of the four health practices, are summarized in Tables IV-5. to IV-8. in the form of unstandardized coefficients, F ratios, and their significance tests. Each table shows a separate model. The assumptions of the regression/correlation procedure are that the respondents were randomly sampled, that their responses were independent, and identically distributed[3] (Kleinbaum and Kupper, 1978).

In Table IV-5. we see the association of religious involvement with the tendency to be overweight. Religious involvement is associated less with being overweight than it is with any of the other health behaviors. After housing stratum and sex are taken into account, only religious preference and knowing one's fellow congregation members are associated with being overweight. People whose religious preference is "Other" emerge as heaviest, as do those who say they know everyone in their congregation. Thus the small association that exists runs counter to the hypothesis that religious involvement will be positively related to the health practice of not being overweight.

The use of alcohol, on the other hand, is associated with three different forms of religious involvement, and in the predicted direction. Table IV-6. shows that after the effects of sex and stratum are considered, the heaviest drinkers are found to be people who have no religious preference, people who say they are only slightly religious, and people who get no strength and comfort from religion. From other models in which sex was included as an interaction term, it can be

Cohesiveness and Coherence

Table IV-5. Unstandardized regression coefficients and
F values for religious involvement and Quetelet Index

	B	F Value
Housing stratum		9.24 *** People in public housing
Public	.287 *	heaviest
Private	-.275 *	
Other	-	
Sex		50.79 *** Males heaviest
Males	.686 ***	
Females	-	
Religious preference		6.67 ** "Others" heaviest
Catholic	.343	
Protestant	.434	
Jewish	-.360	
Other	.613	
None	-	
Religious service attendance		1.63
Never	-.165	
Once or twice a year	.207	
Every few months	-.197	
Once or twice a month	-.106	
Once a week	-.213	
More than once a week	-	
Knowing congregation members		5.20 ** Those who know all heaviest
None	-.584 **	
A few	-.404 *	
Many	-.067	
Almost all	-	
Religious identity		.77
Not religious	-.300	
Only slightly religious	.165	
Fairly religious	.043	
Deeply religious	-	
Strength and comfort		.85
None	.118	
A little	-.132	
A great deal	-	
R^2	.055	

* p < .05   ** p < .01   *** p < .001

Table IV-6. Unstandardized regression coefficients and F values for religious involvement and alcohol use

	B	F Value
Housing stratum		5.60 ** People in "other" housing
Public	-2.858 **	drink most
Private	-1.502	
Other	-	
Sex		195.32 *** Males drink more
Males	9.893 ***	
Females	-	
Religious preference		7.61 *** People with no religious
Catholic	-6.418	preference drink most
Protestant	-7.418 *	
Jewish	-12.042 ***	
Other	-8.796 *	
None	-	
Religious service attendance		1.47
Never	1.527	
Once or twice a year	2.244	
Every few months	-.528	
Once or twice a month	-.929	
Once a week	.801	
More than once a week	-	
Knowing congregation members		.86
None	-1.449	
A few	.020	
Many	.320	
Almost all	-	
Religious identity		6.87 *** People who are slightly
Not religious	-4.523	religious drink most
Only slightly religious	3.177 *	
Fairly religious	2.525 **	
Deeply religious	-	
Strength and comfort		8.70 *** People who get no comfort
None	7.532 ***	drink most
A little	2.089 *	
A great deal	-	
R^2	.123	

* $p < .05$ ** $p < .01$ *** $p < .001$

added that these associations are similar but more pronounced for men than for women. The consistent association of greater religious involvement with lower levels of alcohol consumption is made especially noteworthy by the religious diversity of the population, and the small number of potentially doctrinally-abstinent Protestants. While religious involvement is frequently considered a factor in studies of alcohol use among adolescents (Hadaway, Elifson, Petersen, 1984), these findings suggest it may be a factor for all age groups.

Physical activity is also positively associated with several forms of religious involvement, though the meaning and direction of the association are open to question. After the effects of the more active men and people who live in the community are removed, being physically active is associated with religious preference, with attending religious services frequently, and with knowing many or all of those in one's congregation, as shown in Table IV-7. Oddly, it is the people with no religious preference who are most active, but this is a small group and the relationship may be confounded by age or some other factor. The strongly significant F ratio for religious service attendance is made more substantively significant by the fact that the mean physical activity score increases at every increasing level of religious service attendance, and those who attend services more than once a week are significantly more active than every other group. In other words, when attendance is treated as a categorical variable with six levels, and each level is compared with the mean score for the most frequent attenders, there is a monotonic decrease in the parameter estimate of mean physical activity score at each decreasing level of attendance. Physical activity is also ordinally associated with knowing others in one's congregation, as those who know everyone are significantly more active on average than those who know many, and those who know many are more active than those who know a few, and those who know a few are more active than those who know none at all. The direction of causality in these associations is, of course, questionable, and the extent to which both are dependent on pre-existing health levels again underscores the need to control for health status in the multivariate analyses.

Finally, there are some interesting associations in Table IV-8. of religious involvement with the tendency to smoke. Men in this age group smoke more than women do, but with sex and housing stratum controlled, religious preference, attendance at services, and religious identity all show associations with smoking. Curiously it is not

Table IV-7. Unstandardized regression coefficients and
F values for religious involvement and physical activity

	B	F Value
Housing stratum		13.09 *** People in "other" housing
Public	-.730 ***	most active
Private	-.443 **	
Other	-	
Sex		77.77 *** Males most active
Males	1.067 ***	
Females	-	
Religious preference		5.29 *** People with no religious
Catholic	-2.008 ***	preference most active
Protestant	-2.021 ***	
Jewish	-1.899 **	
Other	-.943	
None	-	
Religious service attendance		10.73 *** People who go more than once
Never	-1.811 ***	a week most active
Once or twice a year	-.909 **	
Every few months	-.756 *	
Once or twice a month	-.656 *	
Once a week	-.621 *	
More than once a week	-	
Knowing congregation members		3.07 * People who know all
None	-.700 **	most active
A few	-.485 *	
Many	-.335	
Almost all	-	
Religious identity		2.38
Not religious	.890	
Only slightly religious	.481	
Fairly religious	.198	
Deeply religious	-	
Strength and comfort		.26
None	-.231	
A little	-.040	
A great deal	-	
R^2	.100	

* $p < .05$ ** $p < .01$ *** $p < .001$

conservative Protestants, but Jews who smoke least. It is those who attend services more than once a week who tend to smoke least, and the tendency to smoke ordinally increases at every decreasing level of attendance. And among the various levels of religious identity, the deeply religious are the least likely to be or have been smokers. These are really very interesting findings suggesting that religious involvement ought to be included in future studies of the determinants of smoking behavior, and underscoring the necessity of controlling for smoking in evaluating associations between religion and health.

So overall, one would say that there is a positive association between greater religious involvement and good health practices or the avoidance of health risk behaviors. And while every different form of religious involvement is associated with one health practice or another, there is a definite contrast between physical activity, which is associated only with the two public forms of religious involvement, and alcohol use, which is only connected to (the absence of) private involvement. This makes smoking all the more interesting because it is associated with both types of involvement. These associations lend credence to the health behavior hypothesis as an intervening mechanism in the relationship between religion and health and necessitate the inclusion of measures of health practices in future analyses.

Religious Involvement and Social Networks

Do the more and less religiously-involved also differ in their social networks? Do they have larger networks, or more intimate ones? Recall from Chapter I the view taken here, that social networks not only integrate and support, but also regulate and constrain. The two public forms of religious involvement, attendance at religious services and involvement in the life of the congregation, are not simply indications of the individual's readiness to accept the benefits of belonging; participation is a moral requirement. The "social" supports the individual but the individual must also support the social. Some of the individual's time, resources, and personal freedom must be sacrificed for the group's very existence.

The feelings of religious identity, and the perception that religion comforts and strengthens, on the other hand, are indicators of the integration function of religion, the measure of benefits received.

Table IV-8. Unstandardized regression coefficients and
F values for religious involvement and smoking

	B	F Value
Housing stratum		2.18
Public	-.074	
Private	-.051	
Other	-	
Sex		128.33 *** Males smoke more
Males	-.352 ***	
Females	-	
Religious preference		12.56 *** Jews smoke least
Catholic	-.022	
Protestant	.028	
Jewish	.315 *	
Other	.228	
None	-	
Religious service attendance		8.45 *** People who go more than once
Never	-.339 ***	a week smoke least
Once or twice a year	-.373 ***	
Every few months	-.318 ***	
Once or twice a month	-.286 ***	
Once a week	-.137 *	
More than once a week	-	
Knowing congregation members		.37
None	-.062	
A few	-.037	
Many	-.023	
Almost all	-	
Religious identity		12.80 *** People who are deeply
Not religious	-.121	religious smoke least
Only slightly religious	-.212 ***	
Fairly religious	-.209 ***	
Deeply religious	-	
Strength and comfort		.50
None	-.044	
A little	.026	
A great deal	-	
R^2	.116	

* $p < .05$ ** $p < .01$ *** $p < .001$

Thus we can examine through the frame of the religious group the two complementary functions of social networks, and raise the purely sociological questions of the functions of several sectors of the social network.

The coefficients and F ratios for the associations of religious involvement and social networks are presented in Tables IV-9. through IV-13. It can be seen immediately that the R^2 statistics for the models are much lower than were those for the health behavior models. Surprisingly, religious involvement explains less of the variation in social networks than it does in health practices.

The most global measure is the size of social networks. After the fact is accounted for that men and people who live in non-age-segregated housing have larger networks, Table IV-9. shows that religious preference, knowing one's congregation, and getting strength and comfort from religion are all associated with the size of one's network. It seems that Protestants, among the religious traditions, have the largest networks. And getting strength and comfort from religion is ordinally related to the size of one's network; the larger the network, the more comfort received. These are moderately significant relationships. But the strongest association, not surprisingly, is with knowing people in one's congregation. Those who know everyone have the largest networks, and the size of the total network decreases as fewer fellow congregants are known. It should be noted that the correlation between these two may be somewhat inflated if a respondent's family, friends, and neighbors, counted in the social network measure, are also members of his or her church or temple congregation.

The social contact measure, the portion of the network with whom the respondent regularly interacts, is also most strongly correlated with knowing others in one's congregation, as shown in Table IV-10. After the fact is taken in account that people who live in non-age-segregated housing have the most contacts, the largest mean number of contacts are reported by people who attend religious services once a week, by respondents who say they know everyone in their congregation, and by people who are fairly religious. Interestingly, while attendance and knowing other members are both positively and linearly related to the number of social contacts reported, it is not the most deeply religious but those in the middle, the fairly religious, who have the most contacts. In fact, the deeply religious also have fewer social contacts than the slightly or not at all religious. This relationship

Table IV-9. Unstandardized regression coefficients and
F values for religious involvement and size of social network

	B	F Value
Housing stratum		7.74 *** People in "other" housing
Public	-1.861 ***	have the largest networks
Private	-.494	
Other	-	
Sex		18.43 *** Males have the largest networks
Males	1.652 ***	
Females	-	
Religious preference		2.67 * Protestants have the
Catholic	-.402	largest networks
Protestant	.116	
Jewish	-1.397	
Other	-2.852	
None	-	
Religious service attendance		2.07
Never	-2.129	
Once or twice a year	-.394	
Every few months	-1.350	
Once or twice a month	-.415	
Once a week	-.884	
More than once a week	-	
Knowing congregation members		13.09 *** People who know all
None	-2.953 ***	have the largest networks
A few	-2.688 ***	
Many	-.161	
Almost all	-	
Religious identity		.32
Not religious	1.072	
Only slightly religious	-.171	
Fairly religious	.087	
Deeply religious	-	
Strength and comfort		4.13 * People who get the most comfort
None	-2.010 *	have the largest networks
A little	-1.303 *	
A great deal	-	
R^2	.059	

* p < .05   ** p < .01   *** p < .001

Table IV-10. Unstandardized regression coefficients and
F values for religious involvement and social contacts

	B	F Value
Housing stratum		15.88 *** People in "other" housing
Public	-3.123 ***	have the most contacts
Private	-1.479 **	
Other	-	
Sex		3.83 * Males have the most contacts
Males	.887 *	
Females	-	
Religious preference		2.33
Catholic	1.389	
Protestant	.349	
Jewish	-.069	
Other	-1.454	
None	-	
Religious service attendance		3.00 * People who attend more than once
Never	-3.974 ***	a week have the most contacts
Once or twice a year	-2.575 *	
Every few months	-3.449 **	
Once or twice a month	-2.649 *	
Once a week	-2.628 **	
More than once a week	-	
Knowing congregation members		13.09 *** People who know all
None	-4.055 ***	have the most contacts
A few	-3.029 ***	
Many	-.391	
Almost all	-	
Religious identity		2.91 * People who are fairly religious
Not religious	1.084	have the most contacts
Only slightly religious	1.096	
Fairly religious	1.475 **	
Deeply religious	-	
Strength and comfort		2.26
None	-1.338	
A little	-1.229	
A great deal	-	
R²	.066	

* p < .05   ** p < .01   *** p < .001

may be confounded by age: recall the steadily increasing proportion of the deeply religious among those few who survive to the oldest ages. The measure of intimacy reflects the number of people the respondent feels "very close to," who can be trusted with personal matters. The analysis in Table IV-11. shows that people in the non-age-segregated housing again have the largest numbers in this sector of their networks. There are no differences between men and women, or between the religious preference groups. The other four forms of religious involvement, however, do show significant associations, although the relationship is not always a linear one. For example, it is people who attend religious services just once or twice a month who report the largest number of intimate ties, as do those who know many, but not all of those in their congregation. On the other hand, both of the private forms of religious involvement are directly related to having a larger number of close ties; both the deeply religious and those who get a great deal of strength and comfort from religion have the largest number of people they can talk things over with.

The number of friends one has, the non-kin sector of the network, bears little association with religious involvement, as Table IV-12. shows. Men have more friends than women, and for a switch, respondents in private housing for the elderly report more friends than those in public or other housing. After these associations are controlled, both religious preference and knowing others in the congregation are significant, but it is people with no religious preference at all who have the most friends. Again this is a small number and age may well be a confounding factor. More predictably, knowing people in one's congregation is directly related to the number of friends one has.

The R^2 statistics for these first four models are rather small; religious involvement simply does not account for much of the variation in these measures of social networks. The R^2 for the model of marital status, shown in Table IV-13., is quite large by comparison, but notice that it is sex and housing stratum with the large F ratios. Men are much more likely than women to be married, and people who do not live in elderly housing are considerably more likely to be married than those who do. Among the religious traditions, Jews are the most likely to be married. Another interesting finding is that the respondents who attend religious services most frequently, more than once a week, are less likely to be married than those who attend once a week, but their marital status is not significantly different from that of those who never

Table IV-11. Unstandardized regression coefficients and
F values for religious involvement and intimacy

	B	F Value
Housing stratum		4.11 * People in "other" housing
Public	-.171	have the most intimates
Private	-.240 **	
Other	-	
Sex		3.03
Males	.134	
Females	-	
Religious preference		1.31
Catholic	.756	
Protestant	.800	
Jewish	.847	
Other	.804	
None	-	
Religious service attendance		2.59 * People who attend once or twice
Never	-.282	a month have the most intimates
Once or twice a year	-.339	
Every few months	-.341	
Once or twice a month	.063	
Once a week	-.304	
More than once a week	-	
Knowing congregation members		3.20 * People who know all
None	-.161	have the most intimates
A few	.013	
Many	.190	
Almost all	-	
Religious identity		7.87 *** People who are deeply religious
Not religious	.011	have the most intimates
Only slightly religious	-.513 ***	
Fairly religious	-.361 ***	
Deeply religious	-	
Strength and comfort		4.06 * People who get the most comfort
None	-.520 *	have the most intimates
A little	-.200 *	
A great deal	-	

R^2 .042

* $p < .05$ ** $p < .01$ *** $p < .001$

Table IV-12. Unstandardized regression coefficients and
F values for religious involvement and friends

	B	F Value
Housing stratum		4.39 * People in private housing
Public	-.923 *	have the most friends
Private	.207	
Other	-	
Sex		6.88 ** Males have the most friends
Males	.791 **	
Females	-	
Religious preference		4.99 *** People with no religious preference
Catholic	-2.152	have the most friends
Protestant	-1.424	
Jewish	-3.241 *	
Other	-3.918 *	
None	-	
Religious service attendance		1.70
Never	-1.188	
Once or twice a year	.326	
Every few months	-.417	
Once or twice a month	-.358	
Once a week	-.467	
More than once a week	-	
Knowing congregation members		12.67 *** People who know all
None	-2.699 ***	have the most friends
A few	-2.394 ***	
Many	-.647	
Almost all	-	
Religious identity		.08
Not religious	-.184	
Only slightly religious	.058	
Fairly religious	.135	
Deeply religious	-	
Strength and comfort		1.03
None	-.576	
A little	-.554	
A great deal	-	
R²	.043	

* p < .05   ** p < .01   *** p < .001

Table IV-13. Unstandardized regression coefficients and
F values for religious involvement and marital status

	B	F Value
Housing stratum		70.22 *** People in "other" housing
Public	.235 ***	are most likely to be married
Private	.189 ***	
Other	-	
Sex		299.11 *** Males are most likely
Males	-.315 ***	to be married
Females	-	
Religious preference		4.85 *** Jews are most likely
Catholic	-.002	to be married
Protestant	.037	
Jewish	-.097	
Other	-.048	
None	-	
Religious service attendance		3.14 ** People who attend more than once
Never	-.034	a week are most likely to be married
Once or twice a year	-.107 *	
Every few months	-.129 **	
Once or twice a month	-.070	
Once a week	-.099 **	
More than once a week	-	
Knowing congregation members		1.60
None	.062	
A few	.052	
Many	.017	
Almost all	-	
Religious identity		.71
Not religious	.034	
Only slightly religious	-.009	
Fairly religious	-.024	
Deeply religious	-	
Strength and comfort		.26
None	-.034	
A little	-.001	
A great deal	-	
R^2	.205	

* $p < .05$ ** $p < .01$ *** $p < .001$

attend. It is true that women are more likely than men both to attend services more than once a week, and to be widowed, but the relationship persists when sex is controlled.

The most consistent association of religious involvement with the social network measures comes in the form of knowing others in the congregation. But all the other forms of involvement, private and public, are about evenly represented in the models. This lends credence to the theoretical perspective that social networks simultaneously integrate and regulate, make demands and offer support. Most importantly, the overall association of religious involvement with social networks is unquestionably a positive one; higher levels of both public and private religiosity are correlated with larger and more intimate networks as well.

Religious Involvement and the Sense of Coherence

What relationship should religious involvement have to the attributions of meaninglessness and fatalism? The measurement of the meaninglessness construct contains two elements: a "faith that things will turn out all right" and a "sense of belonging." The argument was made in Chapter II that all of the forms of religious involvement should be inversely related to attributions of meaninglessness because they constitute either the existence of, the means to, or the acceptance of, available theodicies.

The analysis summary presented in Table IV-14. indicates that all of the forms of religious involvement are indeed associated with meaninglessness. After taking into account sex and housing stratum, all measures of religiosity are significantly associated at $p < .01$. Again the small number of people with no religious preference exhibit some similarity to the most religious people, by reporting lower perceptions of meaninglessness than any of the religious traditions. But the other associations are just as expected. Those who attend services most, who know everyone in their congregation, and who receive a great deal of strength and comfort from religion also see the most meaning in their situation, significantly more so than every lower level of these forms of religiosity. But there is the recurrent anomaly with the question of religious identity: it is the people who are fairly religious who report the least meaninglessness, although the deeply religious see more meaning in things than those who are not religious at all.

Table IV-14. Unstandardized regression coefficients and
F values for religious involvement and feelings of
meaninglessness

	B	F Value
Housing stratum		7.50 *** People in public housing
Public	-.352 ***	see most meaninglessness
Private	.004	
Other	-	
Sex		2.28
Males	-.120	
Females	-	
Religious preference		4.10 ** People with no religious preference
Catholic	-1.233 **	see most meaning
Protestant	-.985 **	
Jewish	-1.123 **	
Other	-.995 *	
None	-	
Religious service attendance		3.04 ** People who attend more than once
Never	-.562 **	a week see most meaning
Once or twice a year	-.627 **	
Every few months	-.725 ***	
Once or twice a month	-.621 **	
Once a week	-.543 **	
More than once a week	-	
Knowing congregation members		5.13 ** People who know everyone
None	-.558 ***	see most meaning
A few	-.442 ***	
Many	-.402 ***	
Almost all	-	
Religious identity		18.83 *** People who are fairly religious
Not religious	-.328	see most meaning
Only slightly religious	.517 ***	
Fairly religious	.601 ***	
Deeply religious	-	
Strength and comfort		5.47 ** People who get the most comfort
None	-.637 **	see most meaning
A little	-.223 *	
A great deal	-	
R^2	.058	

* $p < .05$ ** $p < .01$ *** $p < .001$

The meaninglessness construct ties together the "meaning" and "belonging" functions of religion. It taps the individual's perception that they belong to a social group, as well as their feelings of hope and optimism about their lives and the future, that "things will turn out all right." Thus the meaning element of the sense of coherence overlaps to a certain extent as an explanatory variable with the integration function of social networks. It thus makes it impossible to draw a sharp line between the coherence and cohesiveness hypotheses at this point, as it was impossible to altogether distinguish between the health behavior and cohesiveness hypotheses in the area of social regulation.

But if religious involvement fosters feelings of *hope*fulness by giving meaning to situations, does it necessarily also mitigate feelings of *help*lessness and fatalism? Could religious involvement be associated with meaning but not with fatalism? Apparently it is. As Table IV-15. shows, except for the fact that people with "other" religious preferences are more fatalistic than Catholics, Protestants, or Jews, none of the other measures of religious involvement have any significant association with fatalism. Although women are more fatalistic than men, and people in public and private elderly housing are more fatalistic than people in non-age-segregated housing, religion has practically nothing to do with fatalism, less, in fact, than it does with any measured health practice or aspect of social network. The finding of no association when one was expected is always awkward, but some attempt at explanation, however speculative, should be made. There were good theoretical reasons for including the fatalism construct in the first place: it has been shown in other research to have a direct association with psychological distress (Wheaton, 1983), and it is closely related to Antonovsky's concept of a sense of coherence (1980). Thus the finding of no association with religious involvement should not be dismissed as random, or as measurement error, or a failure of the theory, but as an empirical finding as worthy of interpretation as any other.

Fatalism, as operationalized here, contains three ideas, or subconstructs: luck, lack of order, and helplessness. Let us take them one at a time. The first item, ("Many things that have happened to me are the result of luck") suggests a lack of individual control over events, without the perception that control is centered anywhere else. There is certainly no hint of divine control. Also, the word luck is used, rather than fate, so even a secular sense of destiny is missing. Thus the religiously involved (one would think) would be unlikely to

Table IV-15. Unstandardized regression coefficients and
F values for religious involvement and fatalism

	B	F Value
Housing stratum		4.79 ** People in public housing
Public	-.326 **	are most fatalistic
Private	-.247 *	
Other	-	
Sex		10.39 ** Females are most fatalistic
Males	.305	
Females	-	
Religious preference		3.80 ** People with "other" religious
Catholic	-.859	preference are most fatalistic
Protestant	-.566	
Jewish	-.903	
Other	-1.296 *	
None	-	
Religious service attendance		1.46
Never	-.373	
Once or twice a year	-.131	
Every few months	-.132	
Once or twice a month	-.292	
Once a week	-.026	
More than once a week	-	
Knowing congregation members		.73
None	.029	
A few	.151	
Many	.173	
Almost all	-	
Religious identity		2.45
Not religious	.462	
Only slightly religious	.252	
Fairly religious	.269	
Deeply religious	-	
Strength and comfort		.89
None	-.208	
A little	.095	
A great deal	-	
R^2	.024	

* $p < .05$ ** $p < .01$ *** $p < .001$

agree with the statement. On the other hand, the word luck has very distinctly positive associations, so if the more religiously-involved had more positive emotional states and tended to focus on the positive events of their lives, they might be more likely to agree. From the lack of association, one must conclude either that there are no such tendencies, or that both are present and they cancel each other out.

The second item calls for another interpretation of biography. ("When I look back I feel my life has had no plan or order to it"). Giving a positive answer to this question strongly implies having thought about it before. So the question is, would the more religious people be more likely to have looked back on their lives than the less religious? One might think that they would be more likely to because religion encourages people to think about their sins, and to interpret the major events of their lives in a religious way. No matter how well or poorly one evaluated one's life, the religious criteria would give an order to it. On the other hand, people with religious beliefs have ready-made interpretations for their lives which they thus never had to be "mindful" about. Perhaps the elderly who are maintaining their areligious stance have made an order for their lives from some other source: a profession, the arts, their ancestors. In this case, it would likely be something they were rather conscious about, because religious involvement is the norm for the elderly. But the results of the analysis indicate, again, that either these tendencies are absent, or both present and nullifying each other.

Finally, the third item asks for an assessment of the individual's present state ("I feel completely helpless"). The assumption may quickly be made that people who have religious resources--whether they are resources of understanding, social support, or whatever--will not feel helpless because they have these resources to fall back on, even (especially) in the most extreme life crises. What may be mistaken about this assumption is the orientation of the helplessness; that is, the religious person may be responding not only to the helplessness they may or may not feel vis-a-vis the external world, but also to the sense of surrender to the Other that is often written about as the core of the religious experience. The religious experience may in fact be characterized as an acceptable, even sought-for, non-threatening feeling of helplessness. But while the emotional content of the experience of religious helplessness may be quite different, the empirical manifestation of helplessness in a psychological scale such as this one could be just the same.

In sum, apparently being religious or not has nothing to do with one's sense of fate, one's perception of order in one's life, or whether or not one feels helpless. In other words, religious individuals cannot be differentiated from non-religious individuals when it comes to issues of personal control. Moreover, this is empirical evidence that helplessness and hopelessness are conceptually distinct. Religious individuals may or may not be helpless but they tend not to be hopeless.

With regard to the analyses of the independent variables in general, the results support earlier hypotheses. With the exceptions of fatalism and the tendency to be overweight, the health behavior, social network, and sense of coherence variables show the theoretically-specified associations. All measured forms of religious involvement have some significant associations, and many of the effects are ordinal across every level of the religion variable. These results support the soundness of the four major hypotheses as possible explanatory factors in the relationship between religious involvement and health. However, while these multiple correlations are meaningful and statistically significant, they are not large and do not threaten the subsequent analyses with multicollinearity. Few of the model R^2 exceed 0.10. The religiously-involved *are* somewhat more likely than the uninvolved to engage in good health practices, to have larger and closer social networks, and to see meaning in their lives. But religious involvement or the lack of it explains a rather small proportion of the variation in health behavior, cohesiveness, and coherence, so they are not likely to make a sufficient explanation for any substantial relationships between religion and health that may be found.

Sex Differences in Religious Involvement, Cohesiveness, and Coherence

This final section examines the relationship of the religion variables with each other, and asks whether these patterns are the same for men and women. While one would expect some correlations between the measures of religious involvement themselves, that must not be assumed. Moreover the patterns should be interesting in themselves, particularly if the men's and women's patterns differ. The goals of the analysis are three: 1) to assess the relative importance of the associations between the various forms of religious activity and belief; 2) to assess the relative importance of the associations between religion, social network size, meaninglessness and fatalism; and 3) to compare the men's and women's patterns.

The statistical technique chosen is log linear analysis (BMDP4F), an attempt to complement the previous multiple regression/correlation analyses with a purely categorical approach (Feinberg, 1980). As described earlier, the technique assesses all possible statistical associations between all variables simultaneously. The statistical assumptions, as for any log linear analysis, are that the respondents to the survey were randomly sampled, that they gave their responses independently, and that their responses were identically distributed throughout the population. The data have a multinomial distribution. The null hypothesis (of independence of responses *within* individuals) would say that, for example, there are no differences in attributions of meaning between people who attend religious services frequently and those who never attend; or that people who know many members of their congregation are no more or less likely to be deeply religious than those who know none.

The maximum number of variables that can be included in this case is seven. This is admittedly a very large number for a log linear analysis but it is possible because the data set is so large.[4] The variables and their possible values are given in Table IV-16.

Table IV-16. Variables included in log linear analysis

NAME	SYMBOL	LEVELS	VALUES
ATTEND	A	3	Never, rarely, often
KNOW	K	2	None/few, many/all
IDENTITY	I	3	Deeply, fairly, not
COMFORT	C	2	Much, little
NETWORK	N	2	0-8, 9+
MEANING	M	2	Hopeful, not
FATALISM	F	2	Helpless, not
SEX	S	2	Male, female

A complete cross-classification of these variables yields a table with 576 cells. Breaking the table down by sex produces two tables with

288 cells each[5]. The tables of observed frequencies are reproduced in Appendix B. In general, one could say that the idea of a log linear analysis is to condense the information of a complete cross-classification into its most essential statistical relationships, producing a model with a likelihood ratio chi square (G^2) that has a probability not significantly different from the chi square of the table as a whole. Because I am interested in all possible relationships in the data, the log linear models are hierarchical; that is, each higher order term includes all the lower-order terms within it. A model with all seven variables in one seven-way interaction would thus contain every possible 6-, 5-, 4-, 3-, and 2-way interaction, as well as all the single terms. This would be called the "saturated" model, and would have a chi square identical to that of the table as a whole. The idea is to find a set of lower-order interactions that will yield expected values in the big table that are not significantly different from the actual values (which would be predicted by the seven-way interaction). The strategy for building the model was to begin with all 2-way interactions, first adding all 3-way interactions in a stepwise manner, and then deleting all 2-way interactions one-by-one.

The final men's model contains 11 2-way interactions (out of a possible 21) and 1 3-way interaction (from a possible 35), but no 4-, 5- or 6-way interactions. It is not significantly different from the saturated model (p > .05).

Model	G^2	df	probability
IF,IM,IN,IC,IA,FN,FAK,MK, NA,NK,CA,CK	284.96	251	.0692

Some indication of the importance of the individual terms in the model as a whole is given by the change (increase) in the model's chi square (G^2) when each term, in turn, is deleted. This ranking of the factors is displayed in Table IV-17. This is a crude measure, meant to suggest general groupings rather than ranks. All the 12 terms are necessary, but the difference each makes to the model varies a great deal.

The final women's model contains four 3-way interactions and four 2-way interactions. While it may at first glance look simpler than the men's model, recall that, in a hierarchical model, each 3-way interaction implies three 2-way interactions in addition to itself, so actually the women's model is more complex. It does not differ significantly from the saturated model (p > .10).[6]

Model	G^2	df	probability
IMN,INA,ICK,FMK,MC,NK CA,AK	269.8	244	0.1225

Table IV-17. Factors in order of G^2 added when deleted from men's model

TERM		G^2	df	probability
[] IC	IDENTITYxCOMFORT	242.09	2	0.0000
() IA	IDENTITYxATTEND	28.64	4	0.0000
() IM	IDENTITYxMEANING	21.94	2	0.0000
() IN	IDENTITYxNETWORK	20.53	2	0.0000
() CA	COMFORTxATTEND	19.94	2	0.0000
() NK	NETWORKxKNOW	14.19	1	0.0000
NA	NETWORKxATTEND	15.37	2	0.0005
FN	FATALISMxNETWORK	10.99	1	0.0009
CK	COMFORTxKNOW	8.03	1	0.0046
IF	IDENTITYxFATALISM	6.95	2	0.0309
FAK	FATALISMxATTEND xKNOW	6.44	2	0.0400

Table IV-18. shows the increase in G^2 when each term is removed singly from the women's model shown above.

In comparing the men's and women's models, the first thing to notice is that the term which emerges as the most important in each model is different. For the men it is the link between religious identity and getting strength and comfort from religion. For the women it is the association between attending religious services and knowing people in the congregation. This is the term that tells more about the arrangement of the values in the table than any other. The two variables are the most closely associated of the seven; they are the ones whose patterns are most closely synchronized among the respondents. The most important term for the men was IDENTITYxCOMFORT, the interpretation of which is that men who say they are deeply religious are the most likely to receive a great deal of strength and comfort from religion, and there is no other group more likely to receive this comfort. The men who are fairly religious are like the men who are not religious in getting little comfort. So for the men the strongest association is between the two private, reflective, solitary, and subjective aspects of religion.

The women are a contrast to this. Their strongest association is ATTENDxKNOW, with frequent attendance most closely associated with knowing many in the congregation. So among the women active social involvement, physical mobility, and willing participation are the influential patterns. Women's religious involvement is thus characterized by its social aspects, and men's involvement is characterized by its private nature.

Table IV-18. Factors in order of G^2 added when deleted from women's model

TERM		G^2	df	probability
[] AK	ATTENDxKNOW	189.11	2	0.0000
() CA	COMFORTxATTEND	37.31	2	0.0000
() NK	NETWORKxKNOW	26.00	1	0.0000
FMK	FATALISMxMEANING xKNOW	9.61	1	0.0019
ICK	IDENTITYxCOMFORT xKNOW	11.44	2	0.0033
INA	IDENTITYxNETWORK xATTEND	15.26	4	0.0042
IMN	IDENTITYxMEANING xNETWORK	10.79	2	0.0045
MC	MEANINGxCOMFORT	7.76	1	0.0053

Looking further, it can be seen that these two most important terms both appear in the model for the other sex but only as part of 3-way interactions. A 3-way interaction means that the relationship between two of the variables depends on the level of the third. IDENTITYxCOMFORT, the important men's term, appears in the

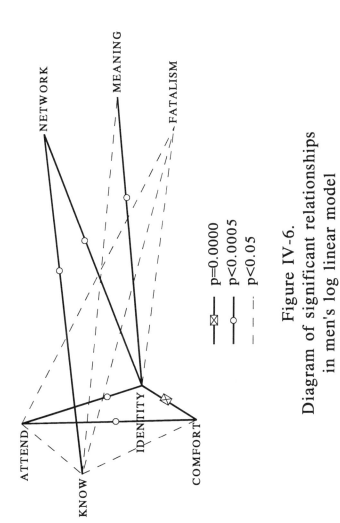

Figure IV-6.
Diagram of significant relationships
in men's log linear model

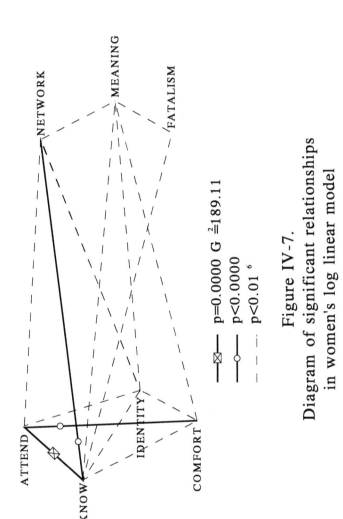

Figure IV-7.
Diagram of significant relationships
in women's log linear model

women's model in an interaction with KNOW; the interpretation of the parameter estimates is that whether or not a deeply religious woman receives a great deal of strength and comfort from religion depends exactly on whether or not she knows a lot of people in her congregation. The most important women's term, ATTENDxKNOW, is in the men's list as part of a three-way interaction with FATALISM. Here, whether or not the men who rarely attend services are fatalistic depends on how many fellow members they know. So both of these interactions are only conditionally significant for the opposite sex.

In the men's model, religious identity stands out as the factor that yields more information than any other. That is, knowing whether or not a man considers himself to be deeply religious tells more about his other religious attitudes and activities, his social network size, and attitudes of meaning and fatalism, than does any other factor in the table. It is present in the first four terms, and in a total of five out of twelve terms, one more than any other factor. There is no such singly important factor for women, attendance and knowing others in the congregation being almost equally important.

Thus far we have looked only at pairs of religion variables. Not surprisingly, the religion variables are more highly related to each other than they are to meaning, fatalism, or social networks. But looking down the men's and women's lists, the first term in which any of the non-religion variables appear bears out the general theme that has been developing, that the social elements of religious involvement are more characteristic of women than of men. The third term in the men's list is IDENTITYxMEANING. The closest link between religion and the non-religion factors for men is thus social-psychological: the tendency is for men who are fairly (*not* deeply) religious to attribute the most meaning to their situation. For women it is the purely social qualities that are most closely linked. The third term in the women's list is NETWORKxKNOW; the more members of her congregation a woman knows, the larger her overall social network is likely to be. The fourth term for both the men and the women is the cross-over term; it links the key characteristic of their religious involvement to the contrasting non-religious factor(s). The term is IDENTITYxNETWORK for men; deeply and fairly religious men are likely to have larger social networks than men who are not religious. The women's term is KNOWxFATALISMxMEANING; women who know many in their congregation are most likely to attribute both fatalism and meaning to their situation, to feel both helpless and hopeful.

Before even the most speculative conclusions regarding these data can be drawn, it should be recalled from the first part of this chapter that women's "religiousness" is stronger than men's on every count, especially in regard to religious identity. While 40 percent of women say they are deeply religious, only 31 percent of men do so. Other differences are similar: 44 percent of women attend services once a month or more, as opposed to 36 percent of men. The log linear analysis, by controlling for all variables simultaneously, shows that the manifestations of women's religious involvement are dominated by their public activities, while men's are primarily organized by private states of consciousness. This means nothing more than that elderly men and women in New Haven exhibit typically different patterns of religious involvement. But importantly, the differences are found to be not only quantitative (which has long been observed), but qualitative.

A question may be raised regarding marital status. The whole difference between men and women could be confounded by marital status differences. It is true that there is a great imbalance: while men are 63 percent married and 23 percent widowed, women are 62 percent widowed and 25 percent married. So if the natural inclination of all bereaved spouses is to attend more religious services, the women will naturally outweigh the men, making the differences due to widowhood and not sex. But from earlier bivariate tables, it can be seen that while widowed women are more likely than expected to attend religious services more than once a week, widowed men are not significantly different from married men when it comes to frequent attendance. Thus while the possibility remains that other, unsuspected factors may be confounding the sex-religious involvement relationships, the most obvious one, marital status, can be discounted.

This chapter has described some of the concrete conditions of the religious involvement of the elderly in New Haven. In contrast to the findings of other studies, active public religious involvement does not show a decline until one looks at the very oldest age groups. On the other hand, private religious involvement remains constant in each age group or increases: the proportion receiving a great deal of strength and comfort from religion is very high and remains steady across the age groups, while the proportion feeling themselves deeply religious rises. These, of course, cannot be considered age effects because of the cross-sectional nature of the data. Nor can they be considered typical of any community other than New Haven, with its particular mix of religious groups and heavy representation of highly observant white Roman Catholics and black Protestants.

The health behavior, cohesiveness, coherence, and theodicy hypotheses all received preliminary support in the sense that they were found to be associated, more or less as predicted, with the various measures of religious involvement. The lack of association of religious involvement with fatalism was unexpected but is in itself a contribution to the understanding of a theoretically important construct.

Finally, the early part of the chapter confirmed the expectation that women would exhibit more religiosity than men. Quantitatively, more women than men of almost every age are religiously involved in every way measured, from behavioral manifestations to pure perception. These findings substantiate and elaborate previous findings. The latter part of the chapter, however, raises some entirely new issues regarding *qualitative* differences in men's and women's religiosity. The finding that the defining features of women's religiosity are social in nature, while men's are more private and subjective must be overlaid with heavy qualifications: the age of the respondents, and the unusual mix of religious and ethnic groups in New Haven alone make generalization impossible. The significance of the finding can only be found in the new questions it raises, but this should not be underestimated given the historical lack of theoretical interest in this area. Further questions regarding sex differences in the functioning of religious involvement may be raised in the analyses of the health measures that follow.

Notes to Chapter IV

[1] As a more "ultimate" value, religion need not appeal to health. On the other hand good health has often been, consciously or unconsciously, considered a sign of grace, as the Mather quotes in the introduction clearly indicate.

[2] "Do you not know that your body is a temple of the Holy Spirit within you, which you have from God? You are not your own; you were bought with a price. So glorify God in your body." (I Corinthians 6:19- 20).

[3] Models were run for men and women separately; with sex as a dummy variable; and with sex in interaction with each religion term. However, the dummy variable models are simplest to report and adequately convey the results.

[4] The practical limit on the number of variables is reached when a cross-classification table of all the variables produces some empty margins and cells with expected values of 0. There are a lot of zero cells in the observed tables (Appendix B), and in such cases it is possible to add 0.5 to all cells. This was not done, however, because none of the expected cells were 0, meaning that there was always something in one margin. The large table and small cells primarily affect the standard errors of the parameter estimates, making them too large, and hence the significance tests for the parameters too conservative.

[5] A combined model for men and women was attempted. It could be done only by collapsing the margins of the table over FATALISM, which had appeared to be the least related factor. The model (including sex and excluding FATALISM) of all 2-way interactions was significantly different from the saturated model, as was the model with all 3-way interactions, and even the model with all 4-way interactions. Thus the loss of a variable and the diminishing of interpretability far outweighed any gain there might have been in a combined-sex model, and the separate models were retained.

[6] Notice that the significance levels chosen for deletion of terms from the men's and women's models are different. To avoid the problems with multiple comparisons inherent in an analysis with so many variables, it is recommended that terms whose significance levels (when deleted from the model) are between .01 and .05 be deleted, and the significance level of the whole model brought as close to .05 as possible without going under. This would apply to the last two terms in the men's model. But when they were deleted the model slipped below .05 so they were retained. The same problem did not occur with the women's model, so all terms greater than .01 are deleted.

V
Chronic Conditions

In this chapter the relationship between religion and the first of the measures of health is examined. The index of chronic conditions is the most highly objective of the measures of health in the study, in that it taps no perceptual or psychological aspects of health. We begin with it, treating it as a dependent variable, and analyzing its association with religious involvement, because it will become a control variable in the analyses of the other measures of health examined subsequently. As will be seen, this chapter is important as much for its results as for its illustration of the logic followed in the analysis.

Method

As described in Chapter III, chronic conditions are measured with an index created by summing up a score for the existence or absence of eleven chronic illnesses or conditions, including myocardial infarction, cerebral hemorrhage, cancer, diabetes, cirrhosis, fractured hip, other broken bones, hypertension, arthritis, Parkinson's Disease, and amputation of a limb. The index is an empiric measure, chosen at the first stages of data analysis, before its associations with any other measures were known. The wisdom of using an unweighted index, in which different aspects of health are apparently confused, may be questioned. Some of these conditions are life-threatening, some are degenerative and have no cure, some imply no risk of mortality but are continually painful and disabling, and some may have been life-threatening or disabling in the past but are now in remission or the individual has recovered from them. The chronic conditions index thus can be considered a general indication of overall health level only, leaving the implications of those conditions, for mortality, disability, etc., unspecified. This measure is highly objective, requiring little or no judgment or interpretation from the respondent.

As such, it becomes a logical way of controlling for objective health status in the next chapter, when analyzing the association between religious involvement and functional disability. In this way a procedure was developed in which each health measure (chronic conditions, functional disability, depression) is first analyzed as a dependent variable, then entered in subsequent analyses as an independent variable. The method followed is a sort of super-hierarchical analysis, in which layers of hierarchical analyses of increasingly subjective health measures are laid over one another, accumulating the impact of the health controls as they progress, and culminating in the analysis of the most subjective indicator of health, the individual's self-assessment.

The analysis of chronic conditions considered alone, then, is a preliminary analysis because it contains no health controls, and hence no way of specifying the question of causal direction in any relationship between religious involvement and chronic conditions. In the second analysis, however, the relationship can be specified by holding constant what could be expected to be the largest correlate of functional disability, chronic illness. Beginning with the analysis of the functional disability index, then, the chronic conditions index becomes an independent variable, and the correlation between religious involvement and chronic conditions can be considered entirely due to the chronic conditions. The same is then true for the analysis of depression, when the chronic conditions and functional disability indices are entered as controls. In the final layer the effects of the chronic conditions, functional disability, and depression, including their associations with religious involvement, are partialled from the respondent's self-assessment of health. This is therefore a very stringent method of controlling for health in the analyses.

Accompanying this unorthodox method for controlling for health is an unorthodox approach to hierarchical regression/correlation analysis. It is customary, in the analysis of psychosocial factors in epidemiology, to control for demographic factors and risk behaviors, the health consequences of which are better known, before the introduction of the psychological or social factors under study. As described in Chapter III, a modified type of hierarchical analysis will be employed here, entering the study variables (the two indices of religious involvement) first, then background demographic factors, then each of the hypothesized intervening factors, and finally the health controls. In this way, suppression effects and indirect effects will be most clearly seen.

Figure V-1. shows the percentage frequency distribution of the scores on the chronic conditions index, adjusted by weighting for sampling design. As one would expect, women report more conditions than men do, 1.85 on average, compared with 1.47, a significant difference (p < .001). Note, however, that this group of elderly people most often reports just 1 or 2 chronic conditions and that substantial numbers of both men and women report none at all. Thus conditions of chronic illness are widespread in this elderly population, but by no means as universal as stereotypes of the ill elderly might lead one to expect.

Results

A preliminary analysis of the bivariate relationships between the two indices of public and private religiosity and chronic conditions revealed no significant relationship with private religiosity (r = .01). There was, however, a significant correlation with public religiosity (r = -.06, p < .01).

Men's Model. A summary of the results of the hierarchical analysis for the men in the sample is presented in Table V-1. The models are to be read down the columns, and the progression of models reads from left to right. The coefficients in the body of the table are unstandardized; those along the right edge are standardized from the final model. The R^2s, their incremental additions to the previous model, and the associated significance tests are along the bottom edge. Categorical variables are treated as a set of (k-1) dummy variables with the mean score of each level tested against the mean score of the last level, the reference group (SAS, 1982). The procedure followed for elimination of variables was this: three variables were retained throughout the analyses regardless of the significance of their coefficients: housing stratum, and the indices of public and private religiosity. Housing stratum was retained, and also entered first because it is the sampling design variable. The two indices of religion were retained because they are the study variables. All other variables were dropped from subsequent models if they failed to reach the p < .05 level of significance. These conditions will remain the same for all subsequent analyses.

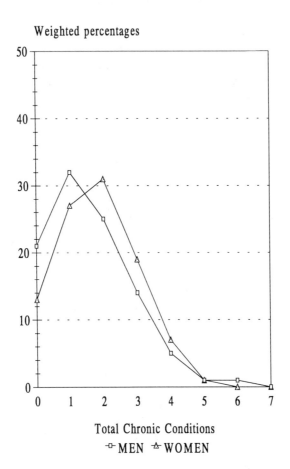

Figure V-1.
Percentage frequency distrubution of men's and
women's total chronic conditions, weighted

The first thing to notice about the men's chronic conditions model is that neither of the two indices of religiosity has a statistically significant coefficient in any of the models. Thus the significant zero-order correlation between chronic illnesses and public religiosity disappears when housing stratum and private religiosity are controlled, and when the sample is limited to men. And evidently no suppression of a true effect is involved. Thus there is no association between men's religious involvement and the number of chronic conditions they report. The following examination of the models one by one serves simply to introduce and illustrate the method that will be followed in the later analyses.

In Model 1, neither of the religion variables are significant, but there is a significant difference in the mean number of chronic illnesses suffered by men who live in public housing when contrasted with those who live in non-age-segregated housing. Men who live in public housing have an average .237 more illnesses than do men who live in "other" housing. The R^2 for the model with three variables is .01; religion accounts for none of the variation in chronic illnesses and housing accounts for almost none.

In Model 2 the background demographic factors are added, age, education, income, and race. None of these variables are significant, nor do they make any change in housing stratum or religion. The R^2 for the model is .02, an insignificant increment over the previous model.

Model 3 introduces the health behavior variable set. As a set, the variables increase the Model R^2 by a significant .03 ($p < .01$), to .05. Moreover, each of the individual variables is significantly correlated with chronic illnesses. For every one unit rise in the Quetelet Index (weight divided by height, squared), there is a .045 rise in the mean number of chronic illnesses suffered ($p < .05$). For every one unit rise in the 14-point activity scale, there is a .045 *decrease* in mean chronic illnesses ($p < .01$). Although these two coefficients are numerically equivalent, they are not comparable because of the different units of the independent variable. When standardized below, however, their relative weights can be compared. A one unit increase in alcohol use (on a 180-point scale) is associated with a .003 ($p < .05$) *decrease* in average chronic illnesses. For smoking, the two categories of present smokers and past smokers were compared with men who had never smoked, and the results show that any smoking at all is

Table V-1. Unstandardized and standardized regression
coefficients for men's chronic conditions models

	Model 1	Model 2 Demog.	Model 3 Health Behavior	Model 4 Cohesive	Model 5 Coherence	Standardized Coefficients Final Model
Stratum: Public	.237*	.234*	.216*	.224*	.223*	.143*
Private	.144	.156	.086	.071	.076	.049
Other[a]	–	–	–	–	–	–
RELIGION						
Public	-.151	-.161	-.038	-.053	-.037	-.014
Private	.022	.028	.048	.048	-.010	-.003
DEMOGRAPHICS						
Age		-.009				
Education		-.006				
Income: $0-4999		-.039				
5000-9999		.042				
10000+[a]		–				
Race: White		-.175				
Black		-.065				
Other[a]		–				
HEALTH BEHAV.						
Quetelet			.045*	.043*	.046*	.076*
Activity			-.045***	-.045***	-.044***	-.113***
Alcohol			-.003*	-.003*	-.003*	-.058*
Smoking: Present			.232*	.231*	.215*	.128*
Past			.348***	.360***	.334***	.199***
Never[a]			–	–	–	–
SOCIAL NETWORKS						
Size				.001		
Contact				.002		
Intimacy				-.016		
Friends				-.003		
Marital: Married				.135		
Ever				.162		
Never[a]				–		
COHERENCE						
Meaning					.018	
Fatalism					-.049**	-.087**
R²	.0104	.0163	.0496	.0513	.0576	
Increment to R²		.0059	.0333**	.0017	.0063	

[a]Reference group
*p < .05   **p < .01   ***p < .001

associated with a higher number of chronic conditions. Men who presently smoke have .232 (p < .05) more average illnesses and men who have quit smoking have .348 (p < .01) more illnesses than men who have never smoked at all. These coefficients are comparable to each other; the higher average number for the past smokers may indicate some recognition of smoking-related health problems by the individuals themselves. In other words, the illnesses may have been the reason for quitting smoking. Indeed one must refrain from imputing any causality in these relationships at all. In particular, being physically active is as likely, maybe *more* likely to be a consequence of illness than it is a measure of prevention. On these grounds an argument could be made for dropping it from subsequent models. However, acknowledging it conservatively as measuring the *ability* to be active, it can serve a useful function as a control variable. The introduction of the health behavior variables reduces the coefficient for housing stratum somewhat, but it remains significant, and the religion variables remain nonsignificant. Thus the health practices are not acting as intervening variables because there is no relationship between religion and chronic illnesses to mediate. Rather they show main effects of their own. They account for a significant amount of the total variation in chronic illnesses that is explained, but it should be emphasized that this is a very small amount, less than five percent.

In Model 4 the social network variables are added. None come close to reaching significance, nor do they cause any changes in any of the other relationships. The R^2 of the model is .05, an insignificant amount larger than the previous R^2. Thus as none of the demographic factors were retained in the analysis, none of the social network measures will be.

The last variables to be introduced are the indicators of meaning and fatalism. There is no significant relationship of chronic illnesses and the attribution of meaning, but there is an association of illness with fatalism. Every unit of increase in fatalism (the lower scores are the more fatalistic) is associated with an increase of .049 average illnesses (p < .01). The amount added to the overall R^2 (.06), is not significant, nor does its inclusion alter the significance of any of the other variables. Fatalism is retained in the final model[1].

The relative importance of the independent variables in the final model can be quickly assessed by scanning the standardized coefficients in the far right column of Table V-1. Smoking is more strongly associated with the number of chronic illnesses a man suffers than is any other factor, and it is the men who have quit smoking who have the largest average number of illnesses. The next largest coefficient is for men who live in public housing, the third for men who presently smoke, the fourth for men who are inactive and fifth for men who are fatalistic.

Summary. There is clearly no support here for the *main hypothesis* of the study, that religious involvement will be positively related to health levels as indicated by the number of chronic conditions a man suffers. There is thus no opportunity to assess the *health behavior*, *cohesiveness*, or *coherence hypotheses* as mediators of the relationship, as there is no relationship to mediate. Some of the variables used to indicate these hypotheses have direct, main effect relationships of their own with chronic conditions; in particular, smoking emerges as the strongest correlate of men's chronic conditions.

Women's Model. The coefficients for the series of women's models are given in Table V-2. It should be immediately noted that these results are quite different from the men's. There is a significant association of the public form of religiosity with fewer chronic illnesses among women, a relationship that is maintained through the entire series of models. Let us examine them one by one.

In Model 1, and for all the models, housing stratum enters first, but has no significant association with women's chronic illnesses. The index of private religiosity is also nonsignificant. However, public religiosity, the summary variable indicating the frequency with which a woman attends religious services, and the proportion of congregation members she knows, is inversely related to the number of chronic illnesses she suffers from. For each one unit change in the 2-point religiosity index, the average number of chronic conditions changes by .211 ($p < .01$). The R^2 for the model is only .01 (F=3.42, df 4, 1503, $p < .01$). The zero-order correlation between chronic illness and public religiosity, then, is probably attributable to the correlation for the women, who make up the majority of the sample. The sex differences in religious involvement thus continue into the health analyses.

Model 2 introduces the demographic factors, age, education, income, and race. Only race is significant; white women have an average .704 fewer illnesses than the "other" women ($p < .01$). Black

Table V-2. Unstandardized and standardized regression
coefficients for women's chronic conditions models

	Model 1	Model 2 Demog.	Model 3 Health Behavior	Model 4 Cohesive	Model 5 Coherence	Standardized Coefficients Final Model
Stratum: Public	.020	.076	-.009	.006	.016	.011
Private	-.027	.020	.002	-.011	.002	.001
Other[a]	–	–	–	–	–	–
RELIGION						
Public	-.211**	-.213**	-.215**	-.224**	-.218**	-.082**
Private	.034	-.005	-.073	-.066	-.059	-.015
DEMOGRAPHICS						
Age		-.006				
Education		.001				
Income: $0-4999		.029				
5000-9999		.089				
10000+[a]		–				
Race: White		-.704***	-.463**	-.462*	-.492*	-.196*
Black		-.290	-.124	-.115	-.158	-.063
Other[a]		–	–	–	–	–
HEALTH BEHAV.						
Quetelet			-.043**	.042**	.043**	.086**
Activity			-.050***	-.052***	-.052***	-.121***
Alcohol			-.006			
Smoking: Present			-.096	-.135	-.126	-.081
Past			.210*	.205*	.184*	.118*
Never[a]			–	–	–	–
SOCIAL NETWORKS						
Size				-.010		
Contact				.003		
Intimacy				.010		
Friends				.009		
Marital: Married				.013		
Ever				.083		
Never[a]				–		
COHERENCE						
Meaning					.032	
Fatalism					-.001	
R^2	.0090	.0328	.0595	.0603	.0583	
Increment to R^2		.0238**	.0267**	.0008	.0000	

[a]Reference group
*$p < .05$ **$p < .01$ ***$p < .001$

women also have fewer average illnesses than "other" women, but the difference is not significant. The introduction of this association does not alter any of the others. It does, however, add a significant increment to the R^2 (.02 added, for a total R^2 of .03).

Model 3 provides the very first example, thus far, of the introduction of one of the explanatory factors into a model with an association between religious involvement and health, and thus the first test of the idea that religion has indirect effects on health via health behaviors. Here in the women's model, as in the men's, there are significant effects among the health behaviors. The Quetelet index is significant (.043, $p < .01$); the heavier a women is, the more illnesses she is likely to have. Physical activity is again strongly inversely related to average chronic illnesses; for every unit increase in the 14-point scale, a woman suffers .05 fewer average illnesses. Women who have smoked in the past, like the men, have more average conditions (.210, $p < .05$) than those who have never smoked, but there is no significant difference between women who still smoke and those who never did. The introduction of the health behavior variables reduces the coefficient for the contrast between white and other women to .463, but it maintains some significance. However, the strength, direction, and significance of the public religiosity index are not affected, in fact the coefficient is just slightly larger. The introduction of the health behaviors adds a significant .03 to the total R^2, making it .06. Thus the health behaviors are apparently not acting as an explanatory factor and mediating the relationship between public religiosity and chronic illness, because they do not diminish it at all. That is, there is no indirect effect. Rather, being overweight, physically active, and smoking have main effects of their own. These factors are retained in the next analyses.

The fourth model brings in the social network variables, and as in the men's model, none are significant. Nor do they alter the R^2 or any of the other associations. Thus the social network variables exhibit no indirect effects or direct effects, and all are dropped from subsequent models.

Model 5 introduces the women's scores for meaning and fatalism. Unlike the men's scores, neither is associated with chronic conditions. Nor do they add anything to the R^2; in fact it actually drops a little because the social network variables are removed. Thus the coherence variables also fail to act as explanatory factors.[2]

Looking at the standardized coefficients in the final column, race, that is, being white, confers the greatest advantage in average number of chronic conditions. The associations of chronic illness with physical activity and having been a smoker are also stronger than with religiosity. But as in the men's model, it must be said that with an R^2 of about .06 this is not a very well-fitting model overall; only a little less than six percent of the total variation in average chronic conditions is accounted for.

To illustrate the magnitude of the association, the index of public religiosity was divided into three roughly equal-sized intervals, and the women were classified as highly, moderately, or not at all involved in public expressions of religious involvement. The regression model was re-estimated using the interval data, permitting a comparison of the mean chronic conditions scores of the most highly and least religious groups. If values are substituted in the equation to represent a white non-smoking woman of average weight, who lives in non-age-segregated housing and engages in moderate levels of physical activity, the model predicts she will report 1.66 chronic conditions if she is highly religious, 1.97 conditions if she is not.

Summary. The analysis of women's chronic conditions supports the *main hypothesis* of a positive association between religious involvement and health. Specifically, it is greater public, not private religiosity that is associated with fewer chronic conditions among women. This association is not in any way "explained" by the *health behavior*, *cohesiveness*, or *coherence hypotheses*, however; while the health behaviors exhibit main effects of their own, they receive no support as an explanatory hypothesis.

Discussion

One may summarize the results by saying that for women, public participation in religious activities is associated with fewer average chronic illnesses. The causal direction of this relationship is left open; without any health controls, the relationship may reflect some selection effect, the simple inability of women with more chronic illnesses to attend religious services. The relatively strong association of chronic conditions and physical activity is another case where the dependent variable possibly affects the independent variable more than the other way around. Physical activity, in the sense of the ability to be active, is retained in the analysis as a control. In a similar fashion, the chronic conditions index will be included in the following analyses as a health control.

A second issue that should be raised is the very low amount of variance accounted for in the two final models, and the doubt this casts on the method of constructing the dependent variable. In order to see if it was the combining of different types of illnesses that caused the models to fit so poorly, three alternative variables were constructed. The first dichotomous variable measured the presence or absence of a life-threatening condition (heart attack, stroke, cancer, or cirrhosis). The second dichotomous variable measured the presence or absence of a non-life-threatening condition (diabetes, broken hip or other bones, high blood pressure, arthritis, amputations, or Parkinson's Disease). A summary index was constructed from these two, made up of four levels: 1) no chronic conditions of any kind, 2) one or more non-life-threatening conditions, but no life-threatening condition, 3) one or more life-threatening but no non-life-threatening conditions, and 4) one or more of each. Bivariate analyses revealed few differences among religious groups for any of the three measures. Multivariate analyses similar to those described in this chapter were performed for the measure of life-threatening conditions[3], and in addition this measure was entered in all the later analyses as a health control. However, as a dependent variable it produced even less well-fitting models than the original chronic conditions index, and as a control variable it removed less variance. Thus on pragmatic grounds alone it could be rejected.

There was a better reason, however, for returning to the original chronic conditions index, despite its flaws. The measure of life-threatening conditions was of some real theoretical interest, which justified the extended investigation it received. The reasoning was that the experience of having suffered an illness of that severity might have religious implications that would not arise in the case of a less serious illness. The results, however, echoed the findings of the Croog and Levine (1972) study of the religious responses of middle-aged male heart attack patients; little or no changes in religious identity were found. And there may be a very good reason for this. The elderly people who report having had heart attacks, strokes, cancer, and liver disease are *survivors* of these serious but survivable illnesses, which may have occurred many years ago. They may, in fact, not be *suffering* from these illnesses at all. Thus the theoretical validity of the variable is seriously compromised by a survivor effect, of which the lack of results is merely an indication, and the original measure of chronic conditions was retained.

In the light of these alternatives and qualifications, then, we can summarize the results of this chapter by saying that *the global hypothesis* of an association between religious involvement and fewer chronic conditions is supported for women, but not for men. Women who are highly involved in the activities of their church or synagogue, who attend services frequently, and who know most or all of the people in their congregation report a lower number of chronic conditions, on average, than do women who are not so involved. This association is not accounted for by the better *health behaviors*, greater *social cohesiveness*, or stronger *senses of coherence* of the religiously-involved women. The analysis of this chapter is primarily important as a groundwork for the following chapters. Only by analyzing chronic conditions first as a dependent variable can one understand exactly what is being partialled out of later analyses.

Notes to Chapter V

[1] The final model can be written as:

$$Y = 1.74 + .22X_{1a} + .08X_{1b} - .04X_2 - .01X_3$$

$$+ .05X_4 - .04X_5 - .003X_6 + .21X_{7a} + .33X_{7b} - .05X_8$$

Where X_{1a} = Public v. "other" housing
X_{1b} = Private v. "other" housing
X_2 = Public religiosity index
X_3 = Private religiosity index
X_4 = Quetelet index
X_5 = Physical activity index
X_6 = Alcohol use index
X_{7a} = Present v. never smoker
X_{7b} = Past v. never smoker
X_8 = Fatalism index

An analysis of the expected values and their residuals reveals no violations of the assumptions of the model. When the residuals are plotted against each of the independent variables, the model is seen to predict equally well (or poorly, more like it) for all groups.

[2] The equation for the final model, then, is:

$$Y = 2.55 + .006X_{1a} + .009X_{1b} - .22X_2 - .05X_3$$

$$- .47X_{4a} - .12X_{4b} + .04X_5 - .05X_6 - .12X_{7a} + .20X_{7b}$$

Where X_{1a} = Public v. "other" housing
X_{1b} = Private v. "other" housing
X_2 = Public religiosity
X_3 = Private religiosity
X_{4a} = White v. "other" race
X_{4b} = Black v. "other" race
X_5 = Quetelet index
X_6 = Physical activity index

X_{7a} = Present v. never smoker
X_{7b} = Past v. never smoker

No violations of the assumptions are revealed by the plots of the expected values and the residuals.

[3]Cleary and Angel (1984) have shown that ordinary least squares and logistic regression produce similar results for dichotomous outcome variables if the positive outcome is found in at least 20 percent and not more than 80 percent of cases. Of the present sample, 31.9 percent had suffered one or more mortal conditions, so it was felt that OLS was justified for this preliminary analysis.

VI
Functional Disability

The ability to function in caring for one's daily needs, of making something to eat, getting up and down the stairs, bathing, and dressing, is the factor that more often than not determines the ability of an elderly person to live independently in their own home. Functional ability, as it is conceptualized here, attempts to measure the capacity of the elderly individual to care for their own basic needs of health and safety without external assistance.

While chronic illness may be the most proximate cause of functional disability in the elderly, there are other important factors as well. Age, sex (Jette and Branch 1981), education, income (Nagi 1976), and race (American Public Health Association 1982) have all been found related to disability. Generally, women, blacks, people over 75, those with little education and the poor suffer the greatest disability and limitations in their daily activity.

The analysis of functional ability is the first opportunity to test an association of religion with some health measure while controlling for another. It is also the first opportunity to test the theodicy hypothesis, that religious involvement may modify the effects of the major determinant of disability, chronic conditions. That is, religious involvement may have a direct relationship with disability, or it may have the effect of diminishing the impact of chronic illness on disability.

Method

The measure of functional disability used in the analysis is a five-point scale constructed from the respondents' replies to questions about fifteen ordinary daily activities. Construction of the index from the three subscales was described in Chapter III.

The first of the three subscales is made up of the seven most basic activities of daily living (Katz, Downs, Cash, and Grotz, 1970). If an individual needed *any* help from a person or equipment, for *any* of the seven items, they received a "1" for the scale. Even with this conservative definition of "ability," 85.5 percent perform all activities with no help. This figure differs somewhat from those of Jette and Branch's (1981) Framingham Disability Study, for several reasons worth pointing out. For six of the seven activities (they did not include using the toilet), Jette and Branch found 96-100 percent of their respondents able to perform "independently," which they also operationalized as not needing help. One reason for difference is to be found in the samples: the Framingham Disability Study surveyed 2654 respondents aged 55-84 years old who were part of the original Framingham cohort, a predominantly white group of middle and upper socioeconomic status. They were thus the survivors of a group that was advantaged in the first place and spanned a younger age range, hence it should not be too surprising that the results are different. Jette and Branch themselves conclude that their population is probably less disabled than the U.S. population.

The second and third subscales (Rosow and Breslau, 1966; and Nagi, 1976) contain eight items tapping mobility and physical ability. The results show fully a third of the respondents, 33.7 percent, able to do all eight activities without any difficulty. Using similar items, but including those with "minimal" difficulty together with those with no difficulty at all, Nagi (1976) found 50.1 percent of his national sample aged 65 and over able to perform all physical activities.

The summary index of functional disability was created by combining these three scales. At one end of the scale are grouped all those who needed any help in even one of the Katz Activities of Daily Living. At the other end are those who needed no help with any of the Katz, Rosow, or Nagi items. And ranging in between are those with some difficulty in one or more of the physical activities. The frequency distribution for this Functional Disability Index is shown in Figure VI-1. These figures are adjusted for sampling design and represent estimated prevalence levels for the elderly population of New Haven. The distribution clearly shows more women at the disabled end of the scale. The women's mean score, 2.67, is significantly higher than the men's 2.18 (p < .001). Again, it should be noted that fully 44 percent of the men and 27 percent of the women are able to perform all fifteen activities, some of which are rather strenuous, without any help or even any difficulty.

The strategy for analysis of the study association and explanatory hypotheses will be the same as in the previous chapter,

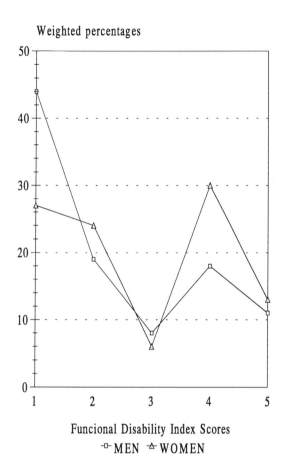

Figure VI-1.
Percentage frequency distrubution of men's and
women's functional disability index scores, weighted

with two important additions. First, by adding the chronic conditions index to the independent variables, it will be possible to look at the relationship of religious involvement and disability both before and after keeping the number of illnesses constant. And second, it becomes possible to assess the theodicy hypothesis by introducing interactions of religious involvement with chronic illness.

Results

The initial bivariate relationship for men and women of functional disability to public religiosity was significant and in the predicted direction ($r = -.19$, $p < .001$). Thus without taking into account any other factors, the more highly involved in the public forms of religiosity a person is, the less likely he or she is to be disabled. Functional disability was not significantly related to private religiosity, ($r = .01$).

Men's Model. A summary of the results of the extended hierarchical analysis are presented in Table VI-1. The format of the table is identical to those in the previous chapter, with the addition of two columns, for the health controls and interactions. Procedures for the introduction and elimination of variables remain the same.

Notice first that the significant relationship of public religious involvement to functional disability is retained across all models, a change from the men's analysis of chronic conditions. It does diminish somewhat as one proceeds across the table, indicating the possibility of some indirect effects, so let us examine the models one by one.

In the first model, containing just the religion indices and controlling for housing stratum, we see that men who live in non-age-segregated housing have less functional disability than men who live in either public or private housing for the elderly. As noted, there is a significant association between greater public religiosity and better functional ability, but apparently there are no differences in functional ability between men who are more and less privately religious. Together, housing stratum and the public religiosity index account for almost 4 percent of the variance in functional disability.

The introduction of the demographic factors in the second model discloses a significant relationship of age and functional ability, a relationship predicted from previous studies. The greater average disability of men in public and private elderly housing is reduced, but still significant. The coefficient for the public religiosity index remains strongly significant, increasing slightly, by .022, from .445 to .467. Overall, the R^2 for the model is .08, a significant increment of .04 over the model that did not include the demographic factors.

The introduction of the health behavior variables again improves the model R^2 significantly, although the reasons for this must be carefully noted. Among the health behavior measures, both alcohol use and physical activity/exercise are positively related to greater functional ability. The relationship of alcohol use to functional disability is oddly opposite to what it should be if abstinence were a preventive health practice, suggesting that, at the cross-sectional level at least, disability tends to reduce consumption of alcohol. More problematic, however, is the positive relationship of physical exercise to functional ability, raising a question about causal direction in the model. Physical activity and functional ability are not measuring exactly the same thing (the R^2 for the entire model is only .17), but functional ability is unquestionably a requirement for the kinds of activities included in the physical exercise measure. On these grounds there would be justification for eliminating it from the model, and in fact in earlier stages of the analysis it was eliminated. On later reflection, however, it was judged more conservative to include it, not as a test of the health behavior hypothesis *per se* but as an additional control on the relationship between public religiosity and functional disability. In fact its inclusion does reduce their relationship; the coefficient for public religiosity in this model is .239, down .128 from that in the previous model but still significant. The major portion of this .128 can be called the indirect effect of public religiosity on functional ability attributable to the greater physical activity of those men who go to religious services often. The remaining .239 is still significant, however, meaning that even within levels of physical activity there is a positive association of functional ability and public religiosity. The borderline-significant coefficient for living in private housing loses significance; age remains strongly significant. Thus while the health behavior variables do not function as expected, they do act as an important control on the relationship of functional ability to public religiosity.

The next model introduces the cohesiveness variables, and finds no significant effects of any of the social network variables. No

Table VI-1. Unstandardized and standardized regression coefficients for men's functional disability models

		Demographics	Health Behavior	Cohesiveness	Coherence
Stratum: Public	.403***	.277*	.234*	.213	.159
Private	.338**	.276*	.154	.134	.120
Other[a]	–	–	–	–	–
RELIGION					
Public	-.445***	-.467***	-.239*	-.281**	-.283**
Private	.077	-.006	-.001	.007	-.025
DEMOGRAPHICS					
Age		.033***	.031***	.027***	.028***
Education		-.023			
Income $0-4999		-.053			
5000-9999		-.057			
10000+[a]		–			
Race: White		-.311			
Black		-.166			
Other[a]		–			
HEALTH BEHAVIORS					
Quetelet			.019		
Activity			-.131***	-.138***	-.132***
Alcohol			-.008***	-.007***	-.007***
Smoking: Present			.073		
Past			.068		
Never[a]			–		
SOCIAL NETWORKS					
Size				.002	
Contact				.001	
Intimacy				-.025	
Friends				-.005	
Marital: Married				.083	
Ever				.045	
Never[a]				–	
COHERENCE					
Meaning					.013
Fatalism					-.077***
HEALTH					
Chronic conditions					
INTERACTION					
Chronic condit.					
No comfort					
A little					
A great deal					
R^2	.0389	.0757	.1708	.1737	.1856
Increment to R^2		.0368***	.0951***	.0029	.0119

[a]Reference group   *p < .05   **p < .01   ***p < .001

Table VI-1. continued

Health	Interaction	Standardized Coefficients Final Model
.101	.101	.055
.092	.097	.053
–	–	–
-.235*	-.233*	-.075*
-.012	-.085	-.023
.032***	.032***	.151***
-.114***	-.115***	-.251***
-.006***	-.006***	-.099***
-.068***	-.067***	-.102***
.363***		
	.426***	.364***
	.383***	.327***
	.344***	.294***
.2826	.2833	
.0970***	.0007	

significant increment is added to the model R^2, and none of the previously significant coefficients are much changed, although public religiosity does increase somewhat. All social network variables are subsequently dropped from the model.

The addition of the coherence variables does add a small increment to the model R^2, making it .19. The meaning variable is not significant, but the fatalism variable is strongly so. The more fatalistic a man is, the more likely he is to also be functionally disabled. Certainly the causal direction is ambiguous. The addition of fatalism to the model has little effect on the coefficients of the other variables. It does not reduce the effect of public religiosity, in fact, it is increased a little bit from the health behavior model, to which the coherence model is most similar. Thus one may not speak of any indirect effect of religiosity on functional ability through the sense of coherence.

In the next model, the measure of chronic conditions is introduced. As expected, it is strongly related to functional disability and increases the R^2 considerably, from .19 to .28. It also slightly reduces the coefficients of nearly all previously significant variables, but all remain significant. In particular, the coefficient for the index of public religiosity is decreased from .283 ($p < .01$) to .235 ($p < .05$). Controlling for health level, then, attenuates, but does not eliminate the tendency for men who are involved in public religious activities to have better functional ability. Part, but not all of the association is due to the fact that the more actively-involved men also have fewer chronic illnesses.

To determine the final model, a series of interactions were tested, pairing chronic conditions with each of the individual religion variables (service attendance, knowing people in the congregation, feeling deeply religious, and getting strength and comfort from religion). The significant interaction is shown at the bottom of the table. When chronic conditions are "nested"[1] in each of the three levels of getting strength and comfort from religion, they have a diminishing association with functional disability as more strength and comfort are gotten from religion. Thus for those men who say they get no strength or comfort from religion, the tendency of more chronic conditions to be associated with greater disability is enhanced. Or in other words, at a given level of chronic illness, men who receive a great deal of comfort from religion will report less disability than men who do not receive such comfort. In the middle are men who receive "a little" comfort, whose estimated coefficient is almost exactly in between the two extremes. Getting strength and comfort from religion is here acting as a "moderator variable" (Cohen and Cohen, 1983) in that it modifies the effect of another variable without itself being related to the dependent variable. The introduction of the interaction has little effect on the other coefficients, and it improves the overall R^2 slightly.

Figure VI-2. shows the relative slopes of the regression lines for the chronic conditions index at three levels of getting strength and comfort from religion. The slopes of these lines are plotted from the final model. That is to say, the graph shows how getting more or less comfort from religion moderates the effects of chronic conditions on disability *when all other factors have been accounted for*. The lines make an ordinal progression, graphically displaying that getting a great deal of comfort from religion reduces the effects of chronic conditions on functional disability by about one third.

Standardizing the coefficients for the final model shows that by far the largest contribution to the explained variance comes from the number of chronic conditions a man suffers, with the men in the category of receiving no strength and comfort from religion being the group with the single greatest risk of disability. The second and third largest amounts come from the effects of chronic conditions at the other two levels of religious comfort. Fourth, fifth, sixth, and seventh are physical activity, age, fatalism, and alcohol use. The main effect of public religious involvement is the smallest of the standardized coefficients.[2]

Summary. The analysis of men's functional disability scores demonstrates very well the analytical advantages of the hierarchical ordering of the variable sets used to test the hypotheses. The *main hypothesis* of the study, that religious involvement will be associated with better functional ability, was supported from the first model to the last, even when levels of chronic conditions were controlled. The direct relationship of functional disability to religious involvement was with the public forms of religious activity, not the private forms.

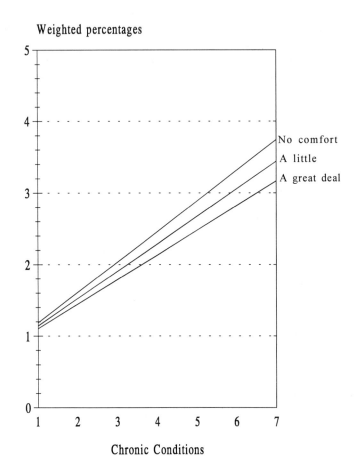

Figure VI-2.
Effect of chronic conditions on men's functional
disability at three levels of religious comfort

The *health behavior hypothesis* is somewhat difficult to assess. While two of the health behavior variables did have significant associations with functional disability, and while the introduction of these variables did reduce the association of religious involvement and disability, it would be hard to argue that this is evidence of better health habits on the part of the religiously-involved. First of all, alcohol use is associated with *better* functional ability. And second, the cross-sectional nature of the data strongly suggest a causal interpretation in which minimal levels of functional ability are preconditions for the activities, making up the physical exercise measure. Thus as an explanatory hypothesis, the health behaviors receive no support.

The *cohesiveness hypothesis* can be more easily dismissed; none of its component variables had any main effects of their own, nor did they diminish the association of religious involvement and disability.

The *coherence hypothesis* also receives no support as an explanatory hypothesis. While fatalism is directly related to disability, it does not account for any of the relationship between religious involvement and disability.

The *theodicy hypothesis*, on the other hand, receives quite strong support from the data. One of the *private* forms of religious involvement, that is, one which requires no physical effort, modifies the way chronic conditions manifest themselves in functional disability. A man who is greatly comforted by religion will be less disabled by his chronic conditions.

The coefficient for public religious involvement in the final model is -.233. This, then, can be considered the estimate for the direct effect of public religious involvement; the total indirect effect can be estimated by subtracting the direct effect from the total effect in the first model (.445 - .233 = .212) (Cohen and Cohen, 1983). Thus, some, but not all of the apparent relationship between better functional ability and greater involvement in public religious activities can be attributed to the greater physical activity and fewer chronic conditions of the men who attend religious services more often. None of it can be attributed to their lower senses of fatalism or their larger or closer social networks. To illustrate the overall effect of religious involvement in the model, public religious involvement was divided into three levels and the model re-estimated with the interval data. If the equation is solved with the values for a man of average age, alcohol use, activity levels, chronic conditions and fatalistic attitudes, who lives in non-age-segregated housing, his score on the five-point disability index will be 1.9 if he is highly religious and gets great comfort from it, 2.4 if he is not religious and gets no comfort.

Women's Model. The results of the analysis of women's functional disability are given in Table VI-2. They are like the men's results in that public religious involvement remains significant throughout, but unlike them in that for the women there is no significant interaction effect of chronic conditions with the propensity to get strength and comfort from religion. Again, the best way to see what happens is to examine the models one by one.

To begin with, women who live in both private and public elderly housing suffer more average disability than women who live in non-age-segregated housing. And the more involved a woman is in the public forms of religiosity, the less likely she is to be disabled. This is a strongly significant relationship. As in the men's model, there is no relationship at all between functional ability and private religiosity. The R^2 for this initial model is .07.

When the demographic factors are entered, controlling for age and income eliminates the differences between housing strata, and these subsequently remain nonsignificant. The older a woman, the more likely she is to be disabled, and white women are less likely to be disabled than "other" women. The addition of these factors increases the R^2 by a significant .08, to .15, but slightly decreases the coefficient for public religiosity.

The inclusion of the health behavior variables again significantly increases the R^2 by .08, to .23, with all the attendant problems of ambiguous causal direction discussed in connection with the men's analysis. Physical activity is strongly associated with functional ability. Being overweight is associated with disability, as is smoking, although it is not the women who presently smoke, but those who have quit smoking who are more likely to be disabled. As it was for the men, higher levels of alcohol use are associated with lower levels of disability. Income, which was just significant in the previous model loses significance. The introduction of the health behavior variables causes the coefficient for race to increase, evidence for a small suppression effect. The coefficient for public religiosity decreases, however, from -.805 to -.582, and the interpretation is clear: part of the association between greater functional ability and greater public religious involvement must be due to the greater physical capacities, lower tendency to smoke, and lower weight of the religiously-involved women.

The introduction of the cohesiveness variables shows again, as it did for the men, that the social network measures have no relationship of their own with functional ability, nor do they modify the relationship of religion and disability. They are thus eliminated from later models.

Entering the coherence variables shows both the measures of meaning and fatalism significantly related to functional disability. The relationship of meaninglessness to disability is the stronger of the two, a relationship that did not exist at all for the men. Women who find more meaning in their situation are less disabled. The measure of fatalism is less statistically significant; the more fatalistic a woman, the more likely she is also disabled. The addition of these two variables does not add significantly to the model R^2, nor does it reduce the relationship of functional ability and religiosity, in fact it increases slightly. Thus functional ability is independently related to a woman's sense of coherence, and this relationship does not in any way account for the association of disability and religious involvement.

Introducing the chronic conditions index as a health control adds a significant .08 to the model R^2, raising it from .24 to .32. It accounts for some of the advantage in functional ability held by white women, those of normal weight, and the physically active; it accounts for all of the advantage of those who drink, and all of the disadvantage of the former smokers. The coefficient for present smokers becomes significant. The introduction of the health control also reduces the coefficient for public religious involvement somewhat, from -.597 to -.529. Thus some of the remaining association between functional ability and religious involvement not accounted for by the greater physical activity of the religiously-involved, is accounted for by their smaller number of chronic illnesses, but not all of it is.

The same list of interactions were tested for the women's model as had been tested for the men's: the chronic conditions index was paired with each of the original individual religion variables. None were found to be both statistically and substantively significant.

When these coefficients are standardized, some comparison can be made. The largest amount of explained variation in a woman's

Table VI-2. Unstandardized and standardized regression coefficients for women's functional disability models

	Demographics	Health Behavior	Cohesiveness	Coherence
Stratum: Public	.365***	-.012	-.057	.030	.032
Private	.208*	.138	.089	.115	.093
Other[a]	–	–	–	–	–
RELIGION					
Public	-.822***	-.805***	-.582***	-.590***	-.597***
Private	.244	-.005	-.056	-.040	-.060
DEMOGRAPHICS					
Age		.048***	.046***	.050***	.049***
Education		-.001			
Income $0-4999		.316*	.115		
5000-9999		.115	-.038		
10000+[a]		–			
Race: White		-.600*	-.714**	-.639*	-.595*
Black		.000	-.251	-.151	-.175
Other[a]		–	–	–	–
HEALTH BEHAVIORS					
Quetelet			.049**	.046**	.048**
Activity			-.141***	-.137***	-.136***
Alcohol			-.007*	-.009*	-.008*
Smoking: Present			.168	.164	.163
Past			.238*	.266**	.239*
Never[a]			–	–	–
SOCIAL NETWORKS					
Size				-.015	
Contact				.003	
Intimacy				.005	
Friends				.012	
Marital: Married				.213	
Ever				.100	
Never[a]				–	
COHERENCE					
Meaning					.074***
Fatalism					-.049**
HEALTH					
Chronic conditions					
R^2	.0748	.1501	.2275	.2255	.2367
Increment to R^2		.0753***	.0774***	-.0020	.0112

[a]Reference group   *$p < .05$ **$p < .01$ ***$p < .001$

Table VI-2. continued

Health	Standardized Coefficients Final Model
.029	.023
.095	.060
–	–
-.529***	-.177***
-.029	-.002
.049***	.213***
-.423	-.147
-.119	-.039
**	**
–	–
.034*	.054*
-.116***	-.232***
-.006	
.193*	
.167	
–	#
.062***	.088***
-.049**	-.085**
.357***	.304***
.3205	
.0838***	

Lost significance in intermediate models

functional ability can be accounted for by the number of chronic conditions she suffers from. Physical activity and age contribute the second and third largest amounts. But after these important but obvious factors are accounted for, public religious involvement has the next most substantial association with functional disability. The other factors in the final model, in order of importance are: race, meaninglessness, fatalism, and being overweight.

Summary. This analysis of women's functional disability scores again supports the *main hypothesis* of the study, that greater religious involvement (and again it is public, not private religious involvement), will be related to better functional ability. Women who are actively involved in their churches or synagogues are substantially less disabled on average than those who are not, even within levels of chronic conditions and ability to be physically active.

Some of this association may be attributed to the better health behaviors of the religiously-involved women. The analysis of women's functional disability supports the *health behavior hypothesis*: some of the association of religious involvement and functional ability may be due to the fact that the religiously-involved women are less likely to smoke, or to have been smokers, a relationship which was detailed in Chapter IV. Other health behaviors provide less evidence of an indirect effect: while the more religiously-active were less likely to consume alcohol, alcohol use is *inversely* related to disability. Being overweight is associated positively with disability, but the problems of causality inherent in the analysis preclude interpreting this as an indirect effect of public religiosity on functional disability through the better exercise habits of the more religious women. Nevertheless, they do smoke less than nonreligious women, and this alone is support for the hypothesis that better health behaviors partially account for the better functional ability of the more religious women.

There is no support whatever for the *cohesiveness hypothesis*. None of the measures have any association with disability. None of the relationship between religious involvement and functional ability can be accounted for by the larger or closer social networks of the religiously-involved.

The *coherence hypothesis* also fails to receive support. In spite of the significant associations of both meaninglessness and fatalism with disability, their addition to the model in no way reduces the effects of public religiosity. There is thus no basis for considering a sense of coherence to be in any way explanatory of the effects of public religiosity on functional disability.

Finally, the *theodicy hypothesis* fails to be supported. None of the interactions tested substantively modified the effect of chronic conditions on functional disability.

The coefficient for public religiosity in the final model is -.529. The reduction from the total effect in the first model is equal to .293 (-.822 - -.529), which estimates the indirect effect of public religiosity accounted for by the better health habits, greater ability to be physically active, and fewer chronic illnesses of the more religiously-involved women. To illustrate the magnitude of the remaining direct effect, the model was re-estimated with interval data for public religiosity. The results predict that a white woman of average age, weight, and physical activity, who lives in non-age-segregated housing, has average scores for fatalism and meaninglessness, and an average number of chronic illnesses, will score 2.3 on the functional disability index if she is highly religiously involved, 3.0 if she is not.

Discussion

Among the most disabled people in the sample, that is, the men and women who need assistance with one or more of the most basic activities of daily living, there are 104 (72 women and 32 men) who attend religious services at least once a month. In addition, the large number overall who need "some" help with these basic activities indicates substantial social support resources in the community, for none of the respondents are institutionalized. All are living more or less independently. The substantial number of disabled people attending services regularly is evidence of that support, as well as a caution against finding disability over-determinative of religious activity.

Jette and Branch (1981) observe that old age is too often considered synonymous with illness and disability. Advancing age does predict functional disability but there are other factors, in their study and in this, that are more important. For men and women, chronic illnesses, and physical activity were more highly associated with functional ability than was age. For both men and women, the factor most associated with functional disability was the number of chronic conditions reported. This was precisely Nagi's (1976) finding, a study which included a similar unweighted sum of unspecified "underlying health conditions," and found it the most closely associated with disability.

Both Nagi (1976) and Jette and Branch (1981) found women more disabled than men, as did the present study. On the scale of 5, with 5 indicating the most severe limitations, women averaged 2.7 and men 2.2, a significant difference. The man most likely to be functionally disabled is a man with several chronic conditions who receives no comfort from religion, who is physically inactive, older, fatalistic, does not drink, and who has little public religious involvement. The most functionally disabled women are those who have several chronic conditions, are physically inactive, older, have little public religious involvement, and have strong senses of both meaninglessness and fatalism.

Two of the study's four explanatory hypotheses received some support from the analysis, the health behavior hypothesis in the case of the women, and the theodicy hypothesis in the case of the men. The *behavioral hypothesis* meets the methodological and statistical requirements for a significant indirect effect in both the men's and the women's analysis, but the causal direction of the most statistically important relationship, that of physical activity and functional ability, is so questionable as to make it useful only as a control variable. The association of smoking with women's disability, given the earlier finding of the more religious women's tendency not to smoke, is quite plausible support for the health behavior hypothesis. The fact that smoking maintains, but then loses its significant effect when chronic conditions are controlled, makes it even more plausible.

The *cohesiveness hypothesis*, as operationalized by these network variables, has no significant effects at all.

The *coherence hypothesis* must also be rejected as a mediator of the relationship between religion and functional ability. The association of fatalism with disability, and this is true for both men and women, does not in any way diminish the pre-existing association of religious involvement with disability; indeed it strengthens it in a minor way. Fatalism and disability have an independent relationship that stands on its own.

The fourth hypothesis is the other which finds support, although it is limited to the men's analysis. The *theodicy hypothesis* proposes that religious involvement will modify the consequences of physical illness by reducing the disability associated with it. Private religious involvement had no direct association with functional disability on its own. When linked with chronic conditions, however, it divides the men into three meaningful categories, within which chronic conditions differ in their effect on disability. Getting strength and comfort from religion by no means eliminates the association of chronic illness and disability; the standardized coefficients for the three groups are still the three highest. The most accurate way of describing the effect is to say that men who get little or no comfort from religion are at greater risk of disability than men who get a great deal of comfort. Notice that the coefficient for the main effect of the chronic conditions index is .363. When the interaction is introduced, the coefficients for the three groups become .344, .383, and .426. As a single group, then, the men tend to fall in between the categories of men who get a great deal of comfort and a little. What the interaction reveals, that would not be seen otherwise, is that men who fail to get any comfort at all are at an increased risk of disability.

This finding is very interesting, but not as important overall as the direct relationship between public religiosity and functional ability, the finding which supports the *main hypothesis* of the study. For both men and women, some of this association was clearly due to the advantages of fewer chronic conditions and greater physical activity among the more religiously-involved. But not all of it, or even most of it was indirect in this way, and the remaining relationship deserves further scrutiny. Certainly the association should be pursued in the follow-up data, where changes in disability can also be measured, but no length of follow-up can completely eliminate selection effects that occurred before data collection began. More precise control variables are required in either case; to be specific, a more disability-related, less mortality-related health status measure than the simple unweighted chronic conditions index should be constructed and controlled for. Only in this way can one compare the variations in disability of people with very similar health problems.

Functional disability is one of the difficult circumstances of old age. It is a measure of trouble. In the sense of daily struggles with tasks that were once much easier, or dependence on others for basic necessities, it indicates suffering. It also carries the implication of past suffering, from illnesses or conditions that have left individuals incapacitated in one way or another. At the same time it can claim substantial objectivity as a reliable measure of very basic physical functions, which lends substantive significance to its associations with the psychosocial factors of religious involvement, fatalism, and meaninglessness. The examination of psychosocial factors in functional disability among the elderly is just beginning. The results of this analysis strongly suggest that psychosocial factors may indeed play a role, and that religious involvement in particular, in both its public and private forms, deserves further study.

Notes for Chapter VI

[1] In SAS, when a continuous variable nests with a class variable, the design columns are constructed by multiplying the continuous values into the design columns for the class effect, producing a model which estimates a separate slope for any continuous variable X within each level of class variable A.

[2] The equation for the final model is:

$$Y = .76 + .10X_{1a} + .10X_{1b} - .23X_2 - .08X_3$$

$$+ .03X_4 - .12X_5 - .01X_6 - .07X_7 + .43X_{8a}$$

$$+ .38X_{8b} + .34X_{8c}$$

Where X_{1a} = Public v. "other" housing
X_{1b} = Private v. "other" housing
X_2 = Public religiosity index
X_3 = Private religiosity index
X_4 = Age
X_5 = Physical activity index
X_6 = Alcohol use index
X_7 = Fatalism index
X_{8a} = Chronic conditions index / No comfort
X_{8b} = Chronic conditions index / A little comfort
X_{8c} = Chronic conditions index / A great deal of comfort

An analysis of the expected values and their residuals reveals no violations of the assumptions of the model; a plot of the predicted values against the residual values yields an even, random pattern. When the residuals are plotted against each of the independent variables, the model is seen to predict approximately equally well for all groups, although it predicts especially well for men with five or more chronic conditions, and men who are very active.

[2] The equation for the final model can be written:

$$Y = -.08 + .04X_{1a} + .11X_{1b} - .56X_2 - .01X_3 + .05X_4$$

$$- .44X_{5a} - .12X_{5b} + .03X_6 - .12X_7 + .07X_8$$

$$- .05X_9 + .36X_{10}$$

Where X_{1a} = Public v. "other" housing
$\quad X_{1b}$ = Private v. "other" housing
$\quad X_2$ = Public religiosity index
$\quad X_3$ = Private religiosity index
$\quad X_4$ = Age
$\quad X_{5a}$ = White v. "other" race
$\quad X_{5b}$ = Black v. "other" race
$\quad X_6$ = Quetelet index
$\quad X_7$ = Physical activity index
$\quad X_8$ = Meaning index
$\quad X_9$ = Fatalism index
$\quad X_{10}$ = Chronic conditions index

No violations of the assumptions of the model are revealed by the plots of the expected values and the residuals; the residuals are evenly distributed. The model appears to predict equally well for all groups.

VII
Depression

The study of depression among the elderly leaves one with an interesting paradox. The prevailing theories of the etiology of depression would lead one to predict very high rates among the elderly; as Seligman writes, "The aged are most susceptible to loss of control, particularly in American society; no group, neither black, Indians, nor Mexican-Americans, are in as helpless a state as our aged" (1975, p. 184). Particularly relevant to the elderly is the importance cognitive theories of depression place on the individual's views of the future, depressed individuals seeing the future as ". . . a life of unremitting hardship, frustration, and deprivation" (Beck, 1967, p. 255). Among the things the elderly face in their future are important, uncontrollable outcomes that are as aversive as they are inevitable: bereavement, the loss of friends and siblings, chronic illness, and ultimately their own death. Studies which enumerate these occurrences as life events consistently find them to be more strongly associated with depression than any of the other life events (Paykel et al., 1969; Ayuso-Gutierrez, de Diego, Martin, 1982).

From the perspective of role theory, characteristics of adult sex roles that are alleged to make housewives vulnerable to depression are to a large extent also characteristics of the role of the elderly person: a single, limited role with low prestige that is unstructured and invisible, has unclear, diffuse expectations, and is frustrating to perform (Gove and Tudor, 1973; Rosow, 1974). The fact that so many of the elderly are women and have low incomes, two additional known risk factors, intensifies the expectation of a disproportionately large number of depressed elderly. Thus, according to the theories, depression should be a major problem among the elderly.

And yet epidemiological studies of diagnosed and undiagnosed depression among the elderly show rather consistent results; recent community studies of symptoms of depression, particularly those using the Center for Epidemiologic Studies Depression scale, have found the elderly no more depressed than other age groups, with a tendency to be the least depressed of all. Radloff (1975), with data from Kansas City, Missouri, and Washington County, Maryland, found men and women over age 65 to have the lowest mean scores on the CES-D. Eaton and Kessler (1981), in a national sample, found the highest proportion of those scoring above a cut-off point on the scale to be under age 45, the lowest proportion over 65. Clark et al.'s (1981) study in Los Angeles found that those over 60 scored significantly lower than the younger ages for twelve out of twenty items in the CES-D scale. Finally, and most recently, Haug, Belgrave and Gratton (1984) found no overall change over time in the CES-D scores of a sample of elderly people in Cleveland, Ohio; an approximately equal number of respondents declined and improved during a one-year follow-up period.

Methodological problems which have hindered definitive analyses are the same as those which beset most large-scale epidemiological surveys; in addition, there are some difficulties which pertain specifically to the elderly. For one thing, many of the studies are cross-sectional, making it impossible to disentangle age from cohort effects. If there were a true age effect in depression, it could be decisively demonstrated only in a longitudinal study, where one would expect to see change over time not only as individuals become elderly, but within the elderly group itself. The study of psychosocial factors in depression is particularly plagued by the cross-sectional design; factors such as isolation or inactivity may be the consequences of depression as much as the causes of it.

Other issues specific to the elderly have made the assessment of depression even more problematic. The elderly are often underrepresented in community surveys of the noninstitutionalized population (Weissman and Myers, 1979), and those who are excluded may be precisely those at highest risk of depression. Long interview schedules may tire the elderly respondent more quickly than the younger respondent (Gurland, 1976). Moreover, the use of ostensibly objective symptom scales may conceal some age bias: Clark et al. (1981) found adults over age 60 "quite reluctant" to report that they had crying spells, that their life had been a failure, or that people were unfriendly or disliked them. This suggests that individual items on the CES-D scale may have very different meanings to older and younger individuals, making direct comparisons between age groups less useful. Haug, Belgrave, and Gratton (1984) point out that the somatic symptoms, such as sleep disturbances and feelings of weakness, may well be unusual and indicative of problems for young people, but quite normal for the elderly. Moreover, the elderly may be prone to somatize psychological symptoms that they find socially unacceptable. Some of these methodological issues, then, suggest that depression among the elderly may be underestimated, and some suggest that it may be overestimated, in effect leaving the question an open one. They also suggest that more studies are required of the specific manifestations of depression among the elderly.

Thus contrary to what one would predict from several theories of depression, there is no evidence that the elderly suffer significantly more depression than other age groups. While the present study, being an analysis of data from an elderly population only, cannot address the question of relative depression rates among the different age groups, there are two ways in which it can contribute to the general discussion of depression among the elderly. First, granting that it is subject to all the criticism attached to cross-sectional studies using multidimensional scales, it is a study of a sufficiently large group of elderly that the factor of age *within* the elderly group can be examined, laying the groundwork for future longitudinal studies. The second contribution may come from the lack of fit between the theories which predict high rates among the elderly, and the data that fail to find them. If psychosocial factors are resources in health, that is, if they play a positive role, one might expect to see their protective effects functioning most dramatically in situations where the risks are particularly high, intensifying the importance of factors that may moderate those conditions which are both age-related and depression-related: illness, disability, bereavement. It is a considerably more interesting question to ask why the elderly are not depressed than why they are.

If existing theories of depression are of uncertain value in interpreting available data on depression among the elderly, they have been more useful in looking at sex differences in risk of depression. Surveys using the CES-D scale have consistently found women at increased risk of depression. Eaton and Kessler's (1981) national sample had nearly twice as many women with high scores as men, even when demographic variables were controlled. Clark et al. found a ratio of 1.8 depressed women to 1 depressed man (1981). The tendency of women to score higher on depression symptom scales has led to the general awareness that depression is a special problem for women (Guttentag, Salasin, Belle, 1980; Scarf, 1980). A major interpretation of the finding is that the greater frustrations of women's role(s) "promote mental illness" (Gove and Tudor 1973), and there is some support for this in that men's and women's levels of "psychophysiological distress" have apparently been converging over time (though this may be due more to men's increasing distress than women's improvement), (Kessler and McRae, 1981). There is also support in the finding that men's and women's rates of diagnosed and undiagnosed depression begin to converge after age 55 or 65, when the roles of the two sexes become much more similar (Weissman and Myers, 1979; Gurland, 1976).

For this reason, any sex differences in depression found among the elderly are not so easily interpreted with role theory. More useful is the "extrapolation" of learned helplessness theory outlined in Radloff (1980), in which she argues that women are more susceptible than men to depression because early childhood socialization experiences prevent women from seeing the consequences of their actions on the environment. In adulthood, women have been found to more often attribute their successes to luck or chance rather than their own ability. Additional support for a socialization-based attribution theory is suggested by the fact that men and women exhibit different patterns of symptoms, that women report much more negative affect than men (crying, feeling sad), while men report more irritability (feeling bothered) (Clark et al. 1981); and also by the fact that women's higher rates of depression are balanced by men's higher rates of other psychiatric disorders (Dohrenwend and Dohrenwend, 1976). The present study may contribute to this debate in two ways: in the comparison of men's and women's overall rates of symptomatology in depression, and in the comparison of factors in the men's and women's analysis. Given the literature, one should expect to find higher rates for women and a different set of correlates of depression.

The measure of depression used in the present analysis is the individual's total score on the 20-item Center for Epidemiologic Studies' Depression Scale. The scale was constructed with items chosen from earlier scales and selected to represent all major recognized factors in the clinical syndrome of depression. It has been widely used and extensively validated (Comstock and Helsing, 1976; Radloff, 1977).

As Weissman and Myers (1979) point out, depression can be exhibited as a transient mood; a longer- or shorter-lived symptom; or as a group of persistent symptoms, a syndrome. Each item is scored according to the length of its persistence and/or its presence, and the scores are then summed (the mean of the nonmissing values is substituted for one or two missing values). Higher scores indicate greater depression, or, more properly, *"more reported symptoms of depression"* (Radloff, 1975). A cutoff point of 16 on a scale of 0-60 is commonly used to identify the most depressed, but other investigators have treated the scale as a continuous measure of feelings of depression, reaching results that are reported to be comparable to those reached using the dichotomous measure (Eaton and Kessler, 1981; Radloff, 1975). Given that the present analysis is unweighted for study design and does not have the goal of determining prevalence levels, the scale will be treated as a continuous measurement, which has considerable analytic advantages. It also seems a conceptually sound, even conservative measurement, given the continuity of depression with day-to-day mood changes.

The percentage distribution of CES-D scores for the Yale Health and Aging Project sample, weighted to adjust for study design, is shown in Figure VII-1., (N=2677). Because items were scaled 1 to 4, scores range from 20 to 80, with a mean of 27.9. The distribution is highly skewed. The mean score for the women is 28.7 and the mean score for the men is 26.7; a t-test for the 2-point difference is highly significant (p < .0001). Figure VII-1 shows the general shape of the distributions for the two sexes, the most notable difference being the larger percentage of men reporting no symptoms.

Results

The initial bivariate relationships of both public and private religiosity with the unweighted mean CES-D scores are significant and in the predicted direction. The zero-order correlation of public religiosity and depression score is -.17 (p < .0001); higher public religious involvement is associated with lower depression scores. The correlation for private religiosity is -.06 (p < .0016); again, greater religiosity is associated with lower depression.

Men's Model. Table VII-1. shows the results of the hierarchical analysis of the men's data. The format of the table differs little from that presented in the previous chapter, with the exception of the

Weighted percentages

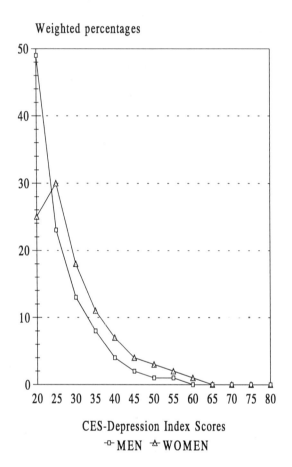

CES-Depression Index Scores
-□-MEN -△-WOMEN

Figure VII-1.
Percentage frequency distribution of men's
and women's CES-D scores, weighted

addition of functional disability to the health controls entered in the analysis in the sixth column.

Looking to the final model last, one can see that public religiosity loses all significant effects when other variables are controlled, but that private religiosity retains a strong relationship with depression until an interaction is introduced. For a clearer understanding of these results, the models should be examined one by one.

In the first model, which introduces just the religion indices and the sampling design variable, all three are significant. Men who live in public housing, on average, score nearly two points higher on the scale than men who live in non-age-segregated housing. Each point on the two-point public religiosity scale is associated with a 1.7-point difference in mean depression scores, and each additional point on the private religiosity scale is associated with a drop of 1.5 points in the average depression score. The R^2 for the simple model is .03.

In the second model, the introduction of the demographic variables causes housing stratum to lose significance, decreases the coefficient and significance level for public religiosity, and increases them for private religiosity. All demographic variables except race are significantly associated with depression scores. Age has a highly significant relationship; for every year older a man is, he gains, on average, .13 points on the depression scale. Income is also highly significant; men whose income is less than $5000 score an average of three points higher than men whose income is over $10,000. Men whose income is between $5000 and $10,000 score two points higher than men with the highest income. Less significant is the relationship of education to depression score; for every additional year of education, a man scores .15 points lower, on average. The R^2 for the model as a whole is increased significantly, to .08. Evidently the differences in mean depression scores between housing strata are accounted for by some combination of differences of the age, education, and income levels of men living in public housing and in the community. Moreover, some of the original relationship between public religiosity and depression is also apparently accounted for by the younger age, or greater education or income of those men who attend religious services frequently, as the introduction of the demographic factors reduces the coefficient for public religiosity from -1.74 to -1.44. At the same time, the coefficient for private religiosity is increased from -1.53 to -2.29, the significance level increasing as well, suggesting that the men who

Table VII-1. Unstandardized and standardized regression coefficients for men's depression models

		Demog.	Health Behav.	Cohesiveness	Coherence
Stratum: Public	1.955**	-.150	-.343	-.585	-.333
Private	.784	.200	-.662	-.590	-.242
Other[a]	–	–	–	–	–
RELIGION					
Public	-1.738**	-1.436*	-1.156*	-.882	-.457
Private	-1.531*	-2.293**	-1.898**	-1.072	-2.209***
DEMOGRAPHICS					
Age		.126***	.101**	.098**	.078*
Education		-.148*	-.093		
Income $0-4999		2.597***	2.685***	2.402***	1.430*
5000-9999		1.996***	2.080***	2.033***	1.132*
10000+[a]		–	–	–	–
Race: White		-2.093			
Black		-1.410			
Other[a]		–			
HEALTH BEHAVIORS					
Quetelet			-.043		
Activity			-.357***	-.343***	-.345***
Alcohol			-.019		
Smoking: Present			1.031		
Past			1.041		
Never[a]					
SOCIAL NETWORKS					
Size				.023	
Contact				-.031	
Intimacy				-.153	
Friends				-.075	
Marital: Married				.793	.075
Ever				2.384**	1.601
Never[a]				–	**
COHERENCE					
Meaning					-.677***
Fatalism					-.795***
HEALTH					
Chronic conditions					
Functional Disability					
INTERACTIONS					
Meaning*Fatalism					
Functional Disability					
Not religious					
Slightly religious					
Fairly religious					
Deeply religious					
R^2	.0353	.0819	.1063	.1066	.1837
Increment to R^2		.0466***	.0244*	.0003	.0771***

Table VII-1. continued

Health	Interaction	Standardized Coefficients
-.657	-.517	-.052
-.469	-.296	-.030
–	–	–
-.035	-.122	.000
-2.221***	-1.129	-.056
.049		
1.439*	1.507*	.145*
1.274*	1.353*	.130*
–	–	–
-.185*	-.187**	-.076**
-.072	-.077	-.007
1.440	1.436	.123
**	**	**
–	–	–
-.670***	-2.771***	-.696***
-.678***	-2.033***	-.575***
.453*	.430*	.068*
1.138***		
	.214***	.659***
	1.701***	.317***
	1.229***	.229***
	1.192***	.222***
	.982***	.183***
.2382	.2529	
.0545***	.0147	

ᵃReference group   *p < .05   **p < .01   ***p < .001

are high in private religiosity are precisely those with lower income, older age, or less education. Controlling for these factors thus removes the suppression effect they were exerting on the relationship of private religiosity to depression.

The health behavior hypothesis may appear less relevant as a factor in depression than in chronic illnesses or functional ability, but the health behavior variables are included here for the sake of completeness. Indeed, none of the measures are associated with depression except physical activity, which as before is as likely to be a cause as a consequence. The measure of activity is strongly related to depression: every one-point increase in the physical activity scale is associated with a .36 drop in mean depression score. This association alone is enough to significantly increase the R^2 for the model as a whole. It also decreases the coefficients for age, and public and private religiosity. Thus another portion of the relationship between public religiosity and depression is accounted for by the greater physical activity of the men who are most religiously involved, and the coefficient is further reduced, to -1.16.

The introduction of the social cohesiveness variables produces a very interesting change in the relationship between the religion indices and depression: when marital status is controlled, both relationships disappear. While there is no significant difference in mean depression scores between men who are presently married and those who never married, men who were formerly married (the majority of whom are widowers) have depression scores that average 2.4 points higher than those of men who had never married. A look back at the analysis of the men's bivariate relationship between marital status and religiosity shows that widowed men are overrepresented in the group that never attends services, and that married men are more likely than expected to know many in their congregation. Thus the relationship between public religiosity and depression that remains when the effects of age, education, income, and physical activity are controlled, is fully explained by the fact that men who have the most public religious involvement are most likely to be married, and least likely to be widowed. In other words, bereavement, or the loss of an important member of the social network is the underlying factor in depression. The disappearance of the relationship between private religiosity and depression is more difficult to explain, because there is no apparent relationship between men's marital status and either form of private religiosity, and because the relationship reappears in the next model.

The addition of the social network variables to the model does not increase the total model R^2.

The addition of the coherence variables, however, does increase the R^2 significantly, from .11 to .18. Both the meaning and fatalism terms are highly significant. A one-point increase in the eight-point meaning scale is associated with a drop of .68 in average depression score. A one-point increase in the twelve-point fatalism scale (the higher score indicating less fatalism) is associated with a .79 drop in average depression score. The introduction of these terms reduces the coefficients for age and income somewhat, but the biggest change is in the measure of private religiosity. Here the meaning and/or fatalism variables are acting as suppressor variables, suppressing some of the variance in depression scores, and thus enhancing the relationship between private religiosity and depression (Cohen and Cohen, 1983). The most plausible interpretation of the finding is that some of the men who are highly privately religious are also somewhat fatalistic, so that when fatalism is controlled the relationship of private religiosity and depression is strengthened.

The introduction of the two health variables again increases the model R^2 by a significant amount, from .18 to .24. An initial effect of controlling for health status is the elimination of the relationship between depression and age, an interesting point in itself, in light of the theories, and suggests that any analysis of depression and aging that fails to take physical health status into account is futile. It also greatly reduces the relationship of physical activity and depression, another indication that physical activity serves, in large measure, as a health status control. Of the two health measures, the functional disability index has the stronger association with depression. For every one-point increase in functional disability, average depression scores rise by 1.14. Every added chronic condition is associated with an increased depression score of .45. The introduction of the health variables reduces the coefficient for the fatalism measure, but the coefficients for meaning and private religiosity stay about the same. Thus physical health status, known to be highly related to depression for all age groups, appears to have a particularly strong relationship to depression in this group of elderly men. It entirely accounts for the apparent tendency for the older men to be more depressed, and also accounts for a portion of the association of depression and the helplessness indicated by the fatalism measure.

To arrive at a final model, a series of interactions was tested. Each individual religion item was paired with each of the two health status measures, and meaning and fatalism were paired with each other. The two interactions which were significant alone and with each other are shown at the bottom of Table VII-1. The interaction of meaning and fatalism is highly significant, as are both of their main effects, whose coefficients are greatly enhanced. Evidently the effect of a combination of certain levels of meaning and fatalism is very strongly related to depression, and suppresses variance that had kept the estimated coefficients for both meaning and fatalism artificially low. The other significant interaction is the modifying effect having a strong feeling of oneself as a religious person has on the association of functional disability and depression. Men who consider themselves not at all religious have an average increase of 1.70 on the depression scale for every unit increase in functional disability. This decreases to 1.23 for men who say they are slightly religious, to 1.19 for men who are fairly religious, and to .98 for men who are deeply religious. The four estimated regression lines are graphed in Figure VII-2., using coefficients from the final model and hence controlling for all other variables. The more religious a man considers himself to be, the more the regression line is pulled toward the horizontal line of no effect. The lines make an ordinal progression; each increased level of religiosity reduces the effect of functional disability on depression. For men who are deeply religious, the effect is only about half of what it is for men who are not at all religious. The decreases are not evenly spread; the biggest difference is between the men who are not religious and those who are slightly religious. The addition of the two interactions increases the R^2 by an almost significant amount. It has little effect on the other coefficients, with the important exception of the main effect of private religiosity, whose coefficient loses significance altogether. Thus the interaction sharpens the analysis by specifying the relevance of private religiosity to the risk of depression among disabled elderly men[1].

The standardized coefficients afford some comparison of the terms in the model. The largest coefficient is for the meaning term, second for the interaction of meaning and fatalism, third for fatalism, fourth, fifth, sixth, and seventh for functional disability at the different levels of religious identity, eighth and ninth for the medium and low income groups, tenth for the widowed men, and eleventh for physical activity. Thus the factors most closely associated with depression in this

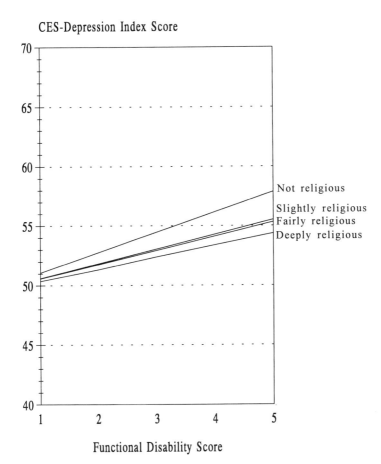

Figure VII-2.
Effect of functional disability on men's CES-D score
at four levels of religious identity

group of elderly men are predominantly psychosocial: their attribution of meaning to their situation, their sense of fatalism, and their functional status in the absence of a religious identity.

Summary. The *main hypothesis* of the study is quite strongly supported by this analysis of men's religious involvement and their reports of depressive symptomatology. For the first time in this study, higher levels of both public and private religious involvement have been related to better health levels, relationships that remained significant even in the presence of demographic factors. The eventual disappearance of the main effect relationships from the final model does not detract from this support since the main hypothesis subsumes the four explanatory hypotheses and all results are in the predicted directions. Greater religious involvement of all kinds is related to lower average levels of depression among elderly men, and the explanatory hypotheses reveal quite a bit about the characteristics of this relationship.

The *health behavior hypothesis* does account for some of the association between religiosity and depression. Physically active men are less likely to be depressed, but as it is not very plausible that their greater religiosity is the source of their activity, there is no real support here for health behaviors as explanatory of the relationship.

The *cohesiveness hypothesis* finds support, in a way, though not the way which might have been anticipated. The marital status of these elderly men entirely and permanently eliminates the association of public religious participation and lower levels of depression. Men who are widowed are more likely to be depressed and at the same time less likely to attend religious services. Whether this can strictly be considered an indirect effect of public religiosity through marital status depends ultimately on the causal ordering (are religiously-involved men more likely to be married, or are married men more likely to be religiously-involved?) but in either case it is an element of social cohesiveness that explains the relationship.

The *coherence hypothesis*, on the other hand, accounts for none of the association between private religious involvement and depression. On the contrary, it strengthens the association. Thus none of the tendency for men who have strong private religious feelings to be less depressed can be attributed to their lower senses of fatalism or meaninglessness.

The *theodicy hypothesis*, however, receives strong support from the analysis, even to the point of eliminating the main effect relationship of private religiosity. Functional disability varies in its association with depression according to a man's sense of religious identity. Dividing the men into these four groups reveals the theodicy function of private religious involvement in a way that the direct association could not. The main effect of functional disability before it is modified by level of religious identity is 1.14, a figure that falls between the coefficients for men who are fairly and deeply religious. The introduction of the interaction reveals the increased risk of depression among men who are functionally disabled and without a sense of religious identity.

To give a sense of the magnitude of the difference in depression scores in men with and without religious involvement, values were substituted in the final model to represent a widower with average income, living in non-age-segregated housing, with average levels of physical activity, an average number of chronic conditions, average scores for meaninglessness and fatalism, and an average level of functional disability. If this man has no private religious involvement and considers himself not at all religious, his predicted depression index score will be 31.6. If he is highly religiously involved and deeply religious, it will be 27.7.

Women's Model. The results of the analysis of the women's depression scores are summarized in Table VII-2. They differ from the men's results in that the final model retains the index for public religiosity, but again there are suppression effects and interactions that can best be looked at one model at a time.

In the first and simplest model, public, but not private religiosity is associated with women's depression scores. The association is highly significant and has a large coefficient: for each unit increase in public religiosity, a woman's average depression score drops by 3.8. There is also a significant difference among housing strata. Women who live in private housing for the elderly score nearly 1.5 points higher than the mean for women in non-age-segregated housing. Together these two factors produce a model R^2 of .04.

In contrast with the men's analysis, only one of the demographic factors is associated with women's depression scores; age, income and race have no effects. Education, however, is highly

Table VII-2. Unstandardized and standardized regression coefficients for women's depression models

	Demographics	Health Behavior	Cohesiveness	Coherence
Stratum: Public	.554	-.137	-.113	-.604	-.349
Private	1.469**	1.350*	.924	.993	1.103*
Other[a]	–	–	–	–	–
RELIGION					
Public	-3.805***	-3.378***	-2.615***	-2.932***	-2.625***
Private	.095	-1.128	-1.290	-.897	-.603
DEMOGRAPHICS					
Age		.010	-.022		
Education		-.315***	-.204*	-.295***	-.123
Income $0-4999		1.373	1.481		
5000-9999		.776	.819		
10000+[a]		–	–		
Race: White		-1.848	-2.579		
Black		-2.365	-3.194		
Other[a]		–	–		
HEALTH BEHAVIORS					
Quetelet			-.068		
Activity			-.400***	-.375***	-.344***
Alcohol			.023		
Smoking: Present			1.159		
Past			.422		
Never[a]			–		
SOCIAL NETWORKS					
Size				.081	
Contact				-.068	-.027
Intimacy				-.188	
Friends				-.090	
Marital: Married				.966	
Ever				1.295	
Never[a]				–	
COHERENCE					
Meaning					-.921***
Fatalism					-.743***
HEALTH					
Chronic conditions					
Functional disability					
R²	.0446	.0658	.0760	.0896	.1589
Increment to R²		.0212**	.0102	.0136*	.0693***

[a]Reference group   *p < .05   **p < .01   ***p < .001

Table VII-2. continued

Health	Standardized Coefficients Final Model
-.473	-.043
.964*	.089
–	–
-1.529**	-.079**
-.829	-.030
-.146*	-.046*
-1.140***	-.249***
-.704***	-.187***
.731***	.100***
1.459***	.238***
.2361	
.0772***	

significant. For every additional year of education a woman reports, her depression score declines by .32. The addition of education to the model increases the R^2 by .02, a significant amount. The coefficients for public religiosity and living in private housing are decreased a bit, suggesting perhaps some higher educational levels on the part of women who live in non-age-segregated housing and who attend religious services frequently.

The addition of the health behavior variables produces a significant association of depression scores with physical activity, as it did for the men. For every one-point increase in the physical activity scale, a woman's depression score drops an average of .40. The addition of physical activity to the model does not add a significant amount to the overall R^2 but it does diminish the coefficients for both public religiosity and education. A portion of the evident relationship between greater public religiosity and lower depression scores must be attributed to the greater physical activity of the most religiously-involved women. Again acting in the capacity of a health status control, physical activity also reduces the relationship between education and depression scores and eliminates the difference between women living in private housing and women living in "other" housing.

The introduction of the cohesiveness measures fails to produce any associations of significance. Unlike the men, women show no relationship of marital status to symptoms of depression. Because the social contact measure came closest to reaching significance, (p=.058), and because some changes were registered in the coefficients of the other variables (education and public religiosity both increased), social contact was retained in the next model.

Adding the coherence variables adds a significant increment to the model R^2, raising it from .09 to .16. Both the meaning and fatalism terms are highly significant. A one-unit increase in the meaning scale is associated with a drop of .92 in average depression score, and a one-unit increase in the fatalism scale is associated with a drop of .74. The most noticeable effect on the other coefficients of the introduction of these variables is the elimination of the association with education. Education has been reported in other studies (Eaton and Kessler, 1981) to have a strong inverse association with CES-D scores, a relationship which persisted when numerous other demographic variables were controlled. The present finding, of an apparent indirect effect of education through the increased attribution of meaning, is very interesting, particularly in that it is sex-specific. The introduction of meaning and fatalism also eliminates any prospect of a relationship between social contact and depression. The coefficient for physical activity is very slightly decreased. The small decline in the coefficient for public religiosity is probably not evidence of an indirect effect through a sense of coherence; it simply is a return to the level before the social network variables were introduced.

The next model, which introduces the health controls, does show an indirect effect, however. The coefficient for public religiosity remains significant, but drops from 2.63 to 1.67 when the measures of functional disability and chronic conditions are included. Thus some, but not all of the relationship between depression scores and attendance at religious services that remains when physical activity and the sense of coherence are controlled can be explained by the better physical health of those who attend services often. Both chronic conditions and functional disability have highly significant effects. For every added chronic condition, .72 points are added to a woman's depression score. And for every unit increase in functional disability, 1.79 points are added. The introduction of the health measures reduces the effect of physical activity sharply, in magnitude and significance level, showing again that it largely functions as an imprecise measure of health status. And the health measures have opposite effects on the meaning and fatalism measures, enhancing one and reducing the other. The coefficient for fatalism drops from .74 to .70, indicating as it did for the men, that poor health is a contributing factor to feelings of helplessness among these elderly women. The coefficient for meaning, on the other hand, is increased from .92 to 1.14.

The same list of interactions were tested in the women's model that had been tested in the men's. None were found to be both statistically and substantively significant[2].

Standardizing the coefficients places the largest importance on the effects of attribution of meaning. Functional disability is second, fatalism and chronic conditions are third and fourth. The contribution made to the explained variance by public religiosity is fifth.

Summary. The *main hypothesis* of the study is supported by this analysis of women's religious involvement and their symptoms of depression. The more publicly-involved a woman is in her church or synagogue, the less likely she is to feel depressed, even when all other factors are controlled for. In the women's case it is specifically public, not private religiosity that is associated with depression, a contrast with the men's analysis.

The *health behavior hypothesis* echoes the men's results: physical activity acts as a health control until the controls themselves are introduced, then its association with depression is nearly eliminated. There is thus no support for the health behavior hypothesis as explanatory factor.

The *cohesiveness hypothesis* also fails to be supported. There are no direct or indirect associations of any social network measure with depression among women. Notably, marital status fails to differentiate women with regard to depression.

The coherence variables look at first as if they may be exhibiting their very first example of an indirect effect: the coefficient for public religiosity decreases .31 from the previous model. But it is nearly identical to the coefficient in the health behavior model, before the nonsignificant social network variables were introduced, and thus the loss cannot be considered due to the introduction of the coherence measures. The measures have strong main effect relationships of their own with depression, but the *coherence hypothesis* fails to be explanatory.

The *theodicy hypothesis* also fails to receive any support, another major difference from the men's model. None of the interactions tested demonstrated statistical and substantive significance.

To illustrate the difference public religiosity can make in women's depression scores, the model was re-estimated using interval data for public religiosity. If all other factors are about average, that is, a woman lives in non-age-segregated housing, with an average number of chronic conditions and level of functional disability, and has average senses of meaning of fatalism, her predicted score on the depression index will be 28.9 if she is highly religious, 30.9 if she is not.

Discussion

In many ways, the analysis of symptoms of depression in the sample is the most substantively significant of the four health measures studied. For one thing, the use of a well-known scale facilitates interpretation and comparability with other studies. Being able to compare the results of analyses of known risk factors adds a foundation of credibility to the exploratory investigation of new psychosocial risk factors. Also, coming third in the hierarchy as it does, it reaps the benefits of having two health status controls whose associations with the psychosocial factors in question have already been examined. Thus the evident strength of the association between religious involvement and symptoms of depression in this elderly sample is perhaps the most important finding of the study. Several issues here bear elaboration.

The first is that the significant differences in men's and women's symptom scores that were found at the beginning of the analysis are borne out by the different models that emerged for the two sexes. The man most likely to report numerous symptoms of depression is a man who sees little meaning in life, is fatalistic, functionally disabled with no sense of religious identity, has a low income, and is widowed. But above all he is a man who finds little meaning in his situation. The woman who is most vulnerable to depression is a functionally disabled and fatalistic woman who has little public religious involvement and is also unable to find meaning in her situation. The most obvious differences in the two models are that public religious involvement, the social, ritualistic, participatory aspect of religious involvement appears to protect women against the symptoms of depression, but plays no role at all for men. Rather, it is marriage, or more precisely, not being widowed, that protects men, and accounts for what might have looked like fewer symptoms of depression among men who attend religious services. Men are also more affected by low incomes than women are. One reason public religious involvement may bear more importance for women may be the generally greater religiosity of women, an aspect of the present sample discussed in Chapter IV. Women, particularly older women, are in a rather small minority if they never attend religious services, or deny that they receive any comfort from religion. One would even have to argue for the likelihood of their perceiving themselves as deviant, if only because so many programs and services for the elderly are sponsored by religious groups. On the other hand, it is the private, more psychological aspects of religious involvement that seem to make a difference in men's depression. Going back to the results of Chapter IV, it would appear that the two characteristic features of men's and women's religiosity are precisely the features that are significantly associated with their lower levels of depression. The public, participatory social factors make a difference for the women, and the private, psychological factors make a difference for the men.

With regard to the conceptual hypotheses of the study, the importance of the association between religious involvement and depression would seem to provide the best opportunity thus far for their assessment. First, the questionable evidence for an indirect effect of public religious involvement on depression through the health behavior indicator of physical activity has been noted, and appropriate caveats made. In any case, the *health behavior hypothesis* is less relevant for symptoms of depression than it is for the other physical health measures.

Second, the men's model provides us with the first example of evidence supporting the *cohesiveness hypothesis*. The significant relationship between public religiosity and symptoms of depression absolutely disappears when men's marital status is taken into account, indicating that this social factor fully explains the tendency for men who are highly (publicly) religious-involved to be less depressed. For women there is no support whatever for the cohesiveness hypothesis. While it certainly appears that social elements of religious involvement are of great importance in women's depression, the generic qualities of social networks tapped by these measures are evidently not the relevant features of the involvement.

Nor could one say that the analyses suggest support for the *coherence hypothesis* as an explanation of the relationship of religious involvement and depression. In the women's analysis the introduction of the meaning and fatalism terms caused no changes in the main effects of public and private religiosity. In the men's, they did not reduce the coefficient, as one would see with an indirect effect, but increased it, by acting as suppressor variables. There is thus no evidence that private religious involvement lowers risk for symptoms of depression because it fosters a sense of coherence. While fatalism has a strong direct relationship with depression, and no significant associations with any of the measures of religious involvement, apparently there are some men who are both highly religious and highly fatalistic, so that controlling for fatalism enhances the effects of private religiosity.

Whatever the assessment of the first three hypotheses, the importance of religious involvement for depression among this sample of elderly is seen not only in its direct associations, but also in the way it acts to modify other important factors in depression. The men's analysis provides strong support for the *theodicy hypothesis*. Indeed, the factor religious involvement modifies is precisely the most important health status factor in the model, functional disability. The interactions have the advantage of interpretive specificity since they were tested with the individual religious involvement items. Thus it is specifically those men who say they are not at all religious who suffer the most symptoms of depression due to their functional disability.

The interesting thing about this interaction is that it underscores the importance identity, or a sense of self has for depression. For the men, a strong religious identity moderates the understandable effect physical disability is likely to have on feelings of depression. Other studies have found that health problems elicit more emotion-focused than problem-focused coping (Coyne, Aldwin, and Lazarus, 1981), and that people who have suffered serious accidents or illness suffer least from depression if they are able to recover a new identity for themselves (Andreasen and Norris, 1972; Bulman and Wortman, 1977). It may be that the elderly, suffering slow, but progressive limitations in their physical powers benefit from having a religious or spiritual basis for their sense of self, an identity which would be untouched by physical decline.

Feelings of depression are above all indications of suffering, of pain in the broadest sense. Pain is an absorbing experience, drawing attention toward itself, demanding interpretation and understanding. The analysis in this chapter suggests that religious involvement provides some means for resolution of problems of pain, that public participation in religious activities and having a sense of oneself as a religious person in some way allay suffering, by drawing the individual's attention away from the problem, putting it into a broader context, and making it meaningful.

Notes for Chapter VII

[1] The equation for the final model is:

$$Y = 49.37 - .52X_{1a} - .30X_{1b} - .12X_2 - 1.13X_3$$

$$+ 1.51X_{4a} + 1.35X_{4b} - .19X_5 - .08X_{6a} + 1.44X_{6b}$$

$$- 2.77X_7 - 2.03X_8 + .43X_9 + .21X_{10} + 1.70X_{11a}$$

$$+ 1.22X_{11b} + 1.19X_{11c} + .98X_{11d}$$

Where X_{1a} = Public v. "other" housing
X_{1b} = Private v. "other" housing
X_2 = Public religiosity index
X_3 = Private religiosity index
X_{4a} = Low v. high income
X_{4b} = Medium v. high income
X_5 = Physical activity index
X_{6a} = Presently v. never married
X_{6b} = Formerly v. never married
X_7 = Meaning index
X_8 = Fatalism index
X_9 = Chronic conditions index
X_{10} = Meaning/Fatalism interaction
X_{11a} = Functional disability index/Not at all religious
X_{11b} = Functional disability index/Slightly religious
X_{11c} = Functional disability index/Fairly religious
X_{11d} = Functional disability index/Deeply religious

An examination of the model's predicted values and residuals reveals a possible mild violation of the assumptions of the regression model. A plot of the predicted values against the residuals shows a slight heteroscedastic fan shape, an indication that the assumption of equal variances may be violated. The skewness of the distribution, while not in itself a violation of assumptions, could cause this pattern. To correct for skewness, a logarithmic transformation was performed on the dependent variable and the model was re-estimated. All terms that had been significant in the original model remained so. The interaction of meaning and fatalism was again significant, and when the effects of functional disability were divided by four classes of religious identity, the same ordinal pattern of effects was exhibited. As the assumption of homoscedasticity underlies the validity of the significance tests of the coefficients, and not the estimation of the coefficients themselves, mild departures are usually not considered a serious problem (Kleinbaum and Kupper, 1978). The model does seem to predict better for the men who never married, but the residuals are apparently randomly distributed on the other variables.

[2] The equation for the final model is written:

$$Y = 41.40 - .47X_{1a} + .96X_{1b} - 1.53X_2 - .83X_3$$

$$- .15X_4 - 1.14X_5 + .70X_6 - .73X_7 - 1.46X_8$$

Where X_{1a} = Public v. "other" housing
X_{1b} = Private v. "other" housing
X_2 = Public religiosity index
X_3 = Private religiosity index
X_4 = Physical activity index
X_5 = Meaning index
X_6 = Fatalism index
X_7 = Chronic conditions index
X_8 = Functional disability index

A plot of the predicted and residual values shows no evidence of heteroscedasticity, its shape is cloudlike. Nevertheless, because of the known skewness of the distribution, the depression measure was given a logarithmic transformation and the model was re-estimated. The results were essentially the same; all terms were again significant and the interaction retained its ordinality. The predicted values from the original model appear to be slightly closer for the least religious women, but other than that, the residuals are randomly distributed.

VIII
Self-Assessment of Health

Certainly the most direct and simplest measure of health in the study is the question, "How would you rate your health at the present time?" Unlike the other health variables, which combine measures of numerous lower order characteristics into an indication of a single, higher order characteristic, a request for a self-assessment of health asks the respondent to do the summarizing. The previously analyzed indices of chronic conditions, functional disability, and depression have the advantage of being objective concepts, objective in the sense that one knows what is being measured, at least to the extent that they are summations of known elements. Asking the individual to assess their own health, however, allows only inferential knowledge of the identity of the elements being assessed. Definitions of health and illness are culturally relative, so assessments based on those definitions must also vary in their meaning. For example, cultures which require physical stamina of all members for the day-to-day survival of the group would have different notions of illness and disability than cultures that have the economic resources to permit the care and support of disabled members.

Thus the respondents' own perceptions of their health are the most subjective of the indications of health in the study, and far from being the most straightforward, are the most uncertain with respect to their meaning. This is not to imply, however, that they are for that reason unreliable, in the sense of being randomly inaccurate. In fact, most researchers have found that self-assessments of health agree rather closely with global assessments made by physicians on the basis of physical examinations (Maddox, 1962; LaRue, Bank, Jarvik and Hetland, 1979). Indeed, one longitudinal study found self-ratings of health more predictive of future physician's ratings than physician's ratings were of future self-ratings (Maddox and Douglass, 1973).

There are discrepancies between physician-based measures and self-perceptions of health, but these should not be viewed as errors, by assuming that the physician rating is a standard against which the subjective rating may be evaluated. If self-perceptions of health were only imperfect approximations of the more objective ratings, one would expect the "errors" to be randomly spread through the populations studied. Actual patterns, however, show systematic variation in the incongruities between subjective and objective measures of health. Studies usually report that, among the "deviants," (those who differed from the physician in their assessment), there are many more health "optimists" than "pessimists," by a ratio of 2 to 1 in one study (Maddox and Douglass, 1973), 3 to 1 in another (LaRue, Bank, Jarvik, and Hetland, 1979).

Self-assessments of health have also been found to vary systematically by demographic category, health practices, social network location, and morale, many of the variables in this study. There are, however, no published studies of the relationship between self-assessments of health and religious involvement of which I am aware. This makes it especially important to control for all factors whose relationship with self-assessment has been suggested by previous work.

The self-perception of health has been shown to vary by age. Maddox (1962) found that, among the elderly, the relatively younger were more likely to be pessimistic about their health. Cockerham, Sharp, and Wilcox (1983) argue that people adjust their perceptions and judgments of health in accordance with the aging process, by implicitly or explicitly comparing their own health with that of their age peers. Their Illinois survey of 660 adults showed that most people in the sixth decade of life and after perceived their health to be much better than that of their peers, the majority of younger people feeling their health to be about the same as their peers. This relationship is significant despite the fact that they also found education to be positively related to self-assessments of health, (and older people tend to have lower educational levels), and despite the higher symptom levels of the older age groups. Another survey of 3402 elderly found that, despite more numerous health problems, the elderly over 75 reported better self-ratings of health than the elderly aged 65 to 75 (Ferraro, 1980). This interesting effect may be attributed to a perception of being a survivor, or to a public exaggeration, shared by the elderly themselves, of the illness and disability of the elderly. This preponderance of health optimism among the elderly certainly suggests that some socially shared perception is being tapped.

Self-perceptions of health also vary consistently by sex; women are nearly always reported to have a better assessment of health than men of similar age and physical status (Fillenbaum, 1979; Ferraro, 1980). Mossey and Shapiro (1982) found that, among the respondents who considered their health excellent or good, the women reported more actual health problems. Stoller (1984) also found elderly women suffering greater health impairments than men at a given level of self-assessment. In fact, in Fillenbaum's study, the women who considered their health to be excellent reported *more* average health problems than men who considered their health just good. Again, this suggests that women compare themselves with other women (who have higher symptom levels than men) and see themselves as better off.

Cockerham, Sharp, and Wilcox (1983) found a similar situation among the blacks in their sample, who both reported more symptoms than whites, and more positive assessments of their health. Together these findings underscore the importance of controlling for demographic factors in any analysis of health self-assessments.

There has been some attention to the hypothesis that individuals who practice good health habits will be more likely to assess their health positively. Physical activity was found to be cross-sectionally associated with better self-assessments of health in studies reported by Maddox (1962) and Stoller (1984). Problems of causality are evident here as they were with the correlation of physical activity with the other health measures; objective health status is correlated with both physical activity and subjective assessment of health. Kaplan and Camacho (1983) report an association (also cross-sectional) between poor self-assessment of health and poor health practices overall, among which they included smoking, overweight, insufficient sleep, alcohol consumption, and physical inactivity. This possibility, that an individual's sense of personal health is influenced by their consciously health-oriented activities, deserves further exploration, a sort of "healthy is as healthy does" hypothesis.

Only the most recent studies have begun to examine the relationship of social networks and self-perceptions of health. The Kaplan and Camacho (1983) analysis of the Alameda County data included the Berkman and Syme (1979) Social Network Index, finding a direct relationship between social disconnection and poor self-assessments of health. Stoller (1984) focused specifically on the role of social isolation in perceptions of health. Proposing two alternative theoretical frameworks, she argues first that informal social networks could be positively related to self-perceptions of health because they reduce environmental demands on elderly individuals, increasing their feelings of functional capability. On the other hand, informal assistance could lead to unbalanced exchange relationships, increasing the psychological effects of physical impairments, and thus promoting a poorer assessment of health. The analysis of the data tends to support the latter interpretation; higher levels of functional impairment are associated with higher levels of informal assistance and also poorer self-assessments of health. However, the data are limited by being cross-sectional and drawn from a predominantly rural area of New York State. Further investigations should be longitudinal and not limited to the informal assistance functions of social networks.

Finally, self-assessments of health have been found to vary systematically with measures of morale or depression. Maddox (1962) found past and current depression and low morale to be associated with poor self-assessments of health, regardless of the physician's medical evaluation. Tessler and Mechanic (1978), reviewing results from four studies of quite different populations (industrial workers, students, prisoners, and the elderly), found psychological distress to be the only consistent correlate of perceived health status when physical health status was controlled. Kaplan and Camacho (1983) found a similar association between depression and self-assessments of health. Moreover, Stoller (1984) found that psychological distress had a stronger correlation with poor self-perceptions of health than did even physical or functional status.

The associations found in these studies between self-assessments of health and age, sex, race, education, health practices, social support, and psychological distress, were all associations which remained when physical health status was controlled. They indicate that something more global than simple physical health or functional status is being measured by these individual perceptions. And if they indicate that the way people define health in responding to the question carries a very large subjective element, that element is given consistent meaning by people in similar social locations. At any given level of objectively measured physical health status, women, the most elderly, blacks, those with more education, better health practices, less dependence on others for daily help, and those with better morale will tend to have more optimistic senses of the state of their health, suggesting consistent variations in definitions of what it is that is being evaluated. What is apparently being expressed is an evaluation of health based on a complex of physical, psychological, and social criteria.

The importance of these socially-rooted subjective perceptions for research was originally limited to their approximate comparability with physicians' ratings, and the great appeal of their economy in survey research. Then, almost by accident, it seemed, self-assessments of health were discovered to be highly significant predictors of mortality in follow-up studies, and new interest in the concept has been stimulated. The first report of an association between mortality and self-perceptions of health was that of LaRue, Bank, Jarvik, and Hetland (1979), who found that self-assessments of health predicted five-year survival among the younger respondents in their study. Their sample, however, was small and not randomly selected. Mossey and Shapiro (1982), with a larger, random sample, and longer follow-up, found a stronger association. In their six-year study of 3128 noninstitutionalized elderly Canadians, they found individuals who assessed their health as poor to be almost three times as likely to die as individuals who assessed their health as excellent. More importantly, they found that the association persisted when age, sex, objective health status, and residence were controlled, and that only age was a stronger predictor of mortality. The strength of the association is most dramatically shown in the fact that the "health pessimists" (those who rated their health as fair or poor when their "objective" health status was good or excellent) were *more* likely to die than the "health optimists" who over-rated their objectively poor health. The authors propose four explanations which could account for the association: self-ratings of health may be very finely tuned indicators of physiological changes, more sensitive than diagnoses of already manifest disease processes; they may simply reflect a more healthy lifestyle; they may be an indirect expression of emotional status; or they may reflect a more general positive, optimistic outlook which itself may be protective. The Kaplan and Camacho (1983) study again found a significant association, but was able to go further and test some of the explanations. In the nine-year follow-up of their sample of 6928 adults, men and women who described their health as poor at the beginning of the study were 2.3 and 5.1 times as likely to die (respectively) as were men and women who considered their health excellent. Their further analysis showed that the effects of self-assessment of health on mortality were independent of the effects of health practices, social networks, and psychological status, and in fact were also independent of the effects of physical health status. They conclude that an individual's self-perception of health plays "a singular role" in predicting mortality, a position which accords well with a generalized susceptibility model of disease causation.

Method

The measurement of self-assessed health used in this study is similar to that used in most studies whose results are reported above. In answer to the question, "How would you rate your health at the present time?" respondents could answer excellent (1), good (2), fair (3), poor (4), or bad (5). No explicit comparison of the individual with his or her age peers is called for, but Maddox and Douglass (1973) note that including such comparisons has little effect on the results, presumably because the comparisons are made implicitly.

Longitudinal studies which treat self-assessed health as an independent variable usually collapse the responses into two categories, or make limited comparisons between the highest and lowest levels (Kaplan and Camacho, 1983; Mossey and Shapiro, 1982). Studies which treat perceived health as a dependent variable, as the present analysis does, have tended to be cross-sectional, and have also considered the variable's full range of categories (Cockerham, Sharp, and Wilcox 1983; Stoller 1984; Tessler and Mechanic 1978).

Figure VIII-1. shows the weighted percentage distribution of self-assessed health levels for the men and women of the YHAP sample. Adjusting for sampling design, women have slightly poorer assessments of their health; a t-test for the difference of means was significant ($p < .001$). As in other studies of the elderly, the majority of respondents assess their health as good or excellent.

Results

Initial unweighted bivariate analyses of the relationships of public and private religiosity with self-assessments of health show a significant correlation only with public religiosity. The zero-order correlation for self-assessment of health and public religiosity is -.13 ($p < .0001$). Greater public religious involvement is associated with higher self-assessments of health. There is no correlation with private religiosity.

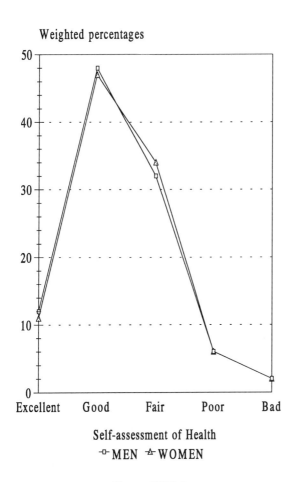

Figure VIII-1.
Percentage frequency distribution of men's
and women's self-assessments of health, weighted

Men's Model. The results for the analysis of men's self-assessments of health are shown in Table VIII-1. The format is identical to those in the previous chapters, except that the measurement of depression is now included as an independent variable.

Scanning the coefficients for public and private religiosity across the models, one immediately sees that neither remain significant through to the final model. Thus one can conclude at the outset that religiosity has no direct relationship to these elderly men's subjective perceptions of their health. Given the zero-order association, however, the development of the hierarchical analysis is instructive.

In the first and simplest model, both public religiosity and housing stratum are significantly associated with men's health assessments. Men who live in public housing have generally poorer assessments of their health than do men who live in non-age-segregated housing. And the more publicly religiously involved a man is, the better his perceptions of his health. In numerical terms, an increase of one point in the public religiosity scale is associated with an improvement of .24 on the health self-assessment scale. The simple model has an R^2 of .03.

The association of public religiosity and self-assessment of health is not changed much by the addition of demographic factors to the model. Controlling for age, education, income, and race does, however, eliminate the significant effect of housing stratum. Among the newly introduced factors, only income is significantly related to self-perception of health. Somewhat surprisingly, given what one would expect from earlier studies, neither age, education, nor race have any relationship to self-perception. Income is not a factor that has been previously reported on in the literature. Self-assessments of health improve as income increases; compared with the highest income category, men in the lowest category score an average .22 points lower in self-assessment. The addition of income to the model increases the R^2 by .02, not a significant amount.

The introduction of the health practice measures does contribute significantly to the variation explained by the model. It also reduces the magnitude and significance level of the index of public religiosity, from -.238 to -.153. Two of the four health practices added to the model have significant associations with self-assessment of health: smoking and physical activity. Men who have quit smoking have poorer self-assessments of their health than men who have never smoked. It is physical activity, however, that has the stronger relationship of the two. Each single point increase in the 14-point physical activity scale is associated with an average .055 improvement in self-assessment. The association between physical activity and perceptions of health repeats earlier findings, and the emphasis on limits in interpreting the causal direction of this cross-sectional association should also be repeated. The finding of an association with smoking is a new one that could be pursued in future studies. It seems clear from these results that some of the association between greater public religiosity and men's better self-assessments of health can be directly attributed to the greater capacity for physical activity and lower likelihood of having smoked of the men who attend religious services more frequently.

The introduction of the social network variables fails to produce any significant associations, nor does it change any of the existing associations. Thus none of the remaining association between public religiosity and men's self-assessments of health can be explained by the effects of larger or more intimate social networks, nor do social networks have any direct relationships with self-assessments of health.

The measures of meaning and fatalism are, however, both directly and indirectly related to self-assessments of health. While the association with fatalism is the stronger of the two, in general, the more meaning a man attributes to his situation, and the less fatalism, the better his self-perceptions of health are likely to be. The introduction of meaning and fatalism into the model eliminates the apparent tendency of men who had quit smoking to evaluate their health more negatively. One might speculate that those men who had quit smoking were fatalistic about the health consequences of their earlier habit; while smoking or not smoking is certainly a matter under individual control, the consequences of past actions are not. The association of income and self-assessments of health is curtailed but not eliminated by the addition of meaning and fatalism to the model. Finally, the already-diminished association of public religiosity and self-assessments of health is further reduced. It would seem that a portion of the relationship that remains is accounted for by the fact that men who attend religious services most frequently are also less fatalistic and/or find more meaning in their situation than men who attend less. The introduction of meaning and fatalism into the model rearranges the variance explained, but does not significantly increase the model R^2.

Table VIII-1. Unstandardized and standardized regression coefficients for men's self-assessment of health models

| | | Health | | |
	Demographics	Behavior	Cohesiveness	Coherence
Stratum: Public	.225***	.056	.055	.038	.029
Private	.062	.015	-.058	-.061	-.047
Other^a	–	–	–	–	–
RELIGION					
Public	-.242***	-.238***	-.153*	-.165**	-.128*
Private	.070	.009	.011	.086	.018
DEMOGRAPHICS					
Age		.000			
Education		-.005			
Income $0-4999		.218**	.242**	.229**	.185*
5000-9999		.196**	.203**	.199**	.160*
10000+^a		–	–	–	–
Race: White		-.257			
Black		-.123			
Other^a		–			
HEALTH BEHAVIORS					
Quetelet			.009		
Activity			-.055***	-.052***	-.055***
Alcohol			- 002		
Smoking. Present			.104	.083	.095
Past			.128*	.126*	.112
Never^a			–	–	–
SOCIAL NETWORKS					
Size				.001	
Contact				.002	
Intimacy				-.022	
Friends				-.009	
Marital: Married				.108	
Ever				.139	
Never^a				–	
COHERENCE					
Meaning					-.032*
Fatalism					-.034**
HEALTH					
Chronic conditions					
Functional disability					
Depression					
R^2	.0307	.0493	.1008	.0961	.1060
Increment to R^2		.0186	.0515***	.0000	.0052#

^aReference group   *$p < .05$ **$p < .01$ ***$p < .001$ #Over Health Behavior Model

Table VIII-1. continued

Health	Standardized Coefficients Final Model
-.015	.051
-.073	-.033
–	–
-.086	-.059
.062	.043
.138	
.119	
–	
-.030***	-.116***
-.018	
-.002	
.074***	.106***
.109***	.192***
.025***	.248***
.2281	
.1221***	

The addition of the more objective health measures to the model finally eliminates the remaining association that self-assessment had with public religiosity. All three health status measures are highly significantly related to men's self-perceptions of health. For every additional chronic condition, a man's self-assessment of health is poorer by .07; for every unit increase in level of disability, a man's self-assessment of health is poorer by .11; and for every increase of one point in depression score, average self-assessment of health levels decline by .03. The addition of the health measures affects all of the other significant associations as well. The coefficient for physical activity is reduced by almost half. The coefficients for income lose significance; recall that income was associated with depression for men. Moreover, the effects of meaning and fatalism completely disappear. This should not be too surprising given the strength of the relationships of both meaning and fatalism with depression in men, and fatalism with functional disability. But it does call into question the causal directions of these associations, issues which can only be addressed by longitudinal research. In any case, it is clear that objective physical, functional, and psychological health status is the salient feature in these elderly men's perceptions of their health. The apparent tendencies of men who attend religious services less frequently, who are physically inactive, fatalistic, and see little meaning in life to perceive themselves as being in poor health are wholly or partly due to the fact that, in the objective sense, they are indeed in poor health. The addition of the health measures more than doubles the model R^2.

As in the previous analyses, a series of interactions was tested, pairing each of the individual religion variables with each of the health measures in turn. None were significant.[1]

A comparison of the standardized regression coefficients shows that depression scores are more highly associated with self-assessments of health than any other factor, echoing the results of Tessler and Mechanic (1978) and Stoller (1984). Functional disability is the second most influential factor, followed by physical inactivity and chronic conditions.

Summary. Men's self-assessments of their health have only an indirect relationship with public religiosity, and none at all with private religiosity. The *global hypothesis* of the study is supported; the relationship is in the predicted direction.

The relationship between greater public religiosity and better self-assessments of health is partly accounted for by the *health behavior hypothesis*: men who are more religious are less likely to smoke or have smoked in the past, and to have better self-assessments of health.

The *cohesiveness hypothesis* finds no support in the analysis.

The association between men's public religiosity and their better self-assessments of health, however, is partly accounted for by the higher senses of coherence of the men who are more publicly religious, and partly by their objectively better health levels. This is the first support in the study for the *coherence hypothesis*.

The *theodicy hypothesis* receives no support; no interactions were significant.

The significant main effect association between public religiosity and men's better self-assessments of health remained until the last model, when the chronic conditions, functional disability, and depression measures were introduced. But recall that men's disability had an association of its own with public religiosity, so religiosity and self-assessments of health have indirect relationships through health behaviors, a sense of coherence, as well as actual health levels.

Women's Model. The analysis of the women's models is presented in Table VIII-2. It differs from the men's analysis in that a main effect of religiosity remains, and one form of religious involvement modifies the effects of objective health status on subjective perceptions of health.

In the first model, controlling only for housing stratum, there is a significant relationship between public religiosity and women's self-assessments of health. The more involved a woman is in the public activities of the religious group, the better her opinion of her health is likely to be. Private religiosity is not associated with perceptions of health. The sampling design variable also shows significant differences: women who live in public or private housing for the elderly are both likely to have poorer self-assessments of health than women who live in non-age-segregated housing. The model's R^2 is .03.

The introduction of the demographic factors does not alter association of public religiosity and better self-assessments of health, although these factors do account for most of the differences between the housing strata. The most significant of the demographic factors is income, with the women in the middle and lower income groups both having significantly poorer self-assessments of health than women

Table VIII-2. Unstandardized and standardized regression coefficients for women's self-assessment of health models

		Demograph.	Health Behav.	Cohesive.	Coherence
Stratum: Public	.207***	.091	.079	.103	.120*
Private	.160**	.140*	.116*	.097	.109
Other[a]	–	–	–	–	–
RELIGION					
Public	-.245***	-.248***	-.110*	-.168**	-.145**
Private	.101	.001	.011	.006	.007
DEMOGRAPHICS					
Age		.003			
Education		-.014*	-.008		
Income $0-4999		.264***	.219**	.282***	.219**
5000-9999		.222**	.165*	.219**	.190*
10000+[a]		–	–	–	–
Race: White		-.134			
Black		.019			
Other[a]		–			
HEALTH BEHAVIORS					
Quetelet			-.005		
Activity			-.055***	-.059***	-.054***
Alcohol			-.005*	-.005*	-.005*
Smoking: Present			.119		
Past			-.007		
Never[a]			–		
SOCIAL NETWORKS					
Size				.003	
Contact				-.008*	-.002
Intimacy				-.010	
Friends				.006	
Marital: Married				.133	
Ever				.067	
Never[a]				–	
COHERENCE					
Meaning					-.050***
Fatalism					-.034***
HEALTH					
Chronic conditions					
Functional disability					
Depression					
INTERACTION					
Funct. dis. * Never					
Once/twice a year					
Every few months					
Once/twice a month					
Once a week					
More than once					
R^2	.0292	.0567	.0836	.0983	.1124
Increment to R^2		.0275**	.0269**	.0147	.0141*

Table VIII-2. continued

Health	Interaction	Standardized Coefficients
.083	.075	.073
.082	.086	.084
–	–	–
.027	-.310***	.170***
.014	.018	.007
.171**	.192**	.162**
.159**	.171**	.144**
–	–	
-.020**	-.020***	-.067***
-.002		
-.041***	-.042***	-.097***
-.006		
.089***	.089***	.129***
.125***		
.026***	.026***	.274***
	.201***	.346***
	.162***	.279***
	.145***	.249***
	.096***	.165***
	.074***	.127***
	.077*	.130*
.2814	.2962	
.1690***	.0148	

ᵃ Reference group   *p < .05   **p < .01   ***p < .001

in the upper income group. Education has a small, but also significant effect that is in accordance with results from other studies; the more education a woman has, the better she perceives her health to be. The inclusion of the demographic factors adds a significant increment to the model R^2, raising it from .03 to .06.

The introduction of the health behavior variables in the third model has a result that is similar to, yet even stronger than that in the men's analysis. In the women's model physical inactivity is associated with poorer self-assessments of health, again acting as a health control. Alcohol consumption is related to better self-assessments of health, not worse, as was also found in a previous analysis. Their inclusion reduces the coefficient for public religiosity from -.25 to -.11 (p < .05). Thus a good part of the reason that women who attend religious services perceive their health to be better is that they are more active than women who do not attend services, that is, women who are probably poorer in objective health status as well. The small association of self-assessment with education is eliminated, and the association with income is reduced. The addition of the health behaviors increases the model R^2 by .03, to .08, a significant increase. The addition of the social network variables to the model provides one of the few examples in the study of a significant association between social networks and health. The more social contacts a woman has, the better her opinion of her health will be. The relationship should not be overinterpreted as it is rather small in magnitude: for every additional individual with whom a woman has regular social interactions, her self-assessment of health is increased by an average .008. The introduction of this factor does, however, increase the model R^2 and affect some of the other coefficients. It increases the effects of income, which raises a very interesting issue about social *contact* as an indication of social networks. This apparent suppression effect suggests that the effects of income are intensified because women at lower income levels have more social contacts, offsetting to a certain extent the effects of low income. This runs counter to the impression that social contacts are facilitated by high incomes. The social contact measure also exerts a suppression effect on public religiosity, which is considerably more difficult to understand. Perhaps involvement in religious activities acts to reduce the numbers of the kinds of contact tapped in the social contact measure: visits and correspondence with children, relatives, and friends; alternatively, people without those contacts may seek more frequent religious involvement. A clue may be provided by the fact that the significantly poorer average self-assessment of the women who live in private housing for the elderly, when compared with the women who live in non-age-segregated housing is now no longer different, when social contacts are controlled. This suggests that women who live in non-age-segregated housing have an advantage over women in private elderly housing in their numbers of social contacts, as well as in their self-assessments of health, and that it is women in non-age-segregated housing with both social contacts and religious involvement who are likely to have the best self-assessments of health. Thus one must conclude that the effects of religious involvement are not accounted for by social cohesiveness, but somewhat intensified by it.

The addition of the coherence variables in the next model, however, eliminates the effects of cohesiveness. The measures of meaning and fatalism are both significantly associated with self-assessments of health, in the expected directions. They add a significant increment to the model R^2, reduce the effects of income and public religiosity, and eliminate the effect of social contacts. The coefficients for physical activity and alcohol consumption remain about the same. Thus there is some support for the coherence hypothesis in interpreting the association between public religiosity and better perceptions of health among these women: a portion of the association is due to the greater senses of coherence among the women who attend religious services and perceive their health to be better. Moreover, the entire effect of social contact can be explained in this way.

In the men's model, entering the objective health status measures into the analysis removed the effects of public religiosity, meaning, and fatalism completely. In the women's model the effects of public religiosity are also temporarily eliminated. Thus the relationship remaining between religiosity and self-assessment when physical activity, meaning, and fatalism were controlled can now be attributed to the better objective health status of the women who attend religious services frequently. The health measures, in addition, reduce the coefficients for physical activity and income, though both remain significant, and eliminate the effect of alcohol. As in the men's analysis, the association between fatalism and poorer assessments of health is completely accounted for by the poorer actual health of the fatalistic women. But unlike the results for the men, women who find more meaning in their condition, regardless of the level of objective health status, are likely to be optimistic in their health assessments. The objective health measures reduce the magnitude of this relationship somewhat, but not its significance level. Their inclusion more than doubles the model R^2, making it .29.

As in the other analyses, attempts were made to modify the effects of the strongest correlates of self-assessment with the separate religion variables, and one was found to be significant. When the highly significant effects of functional disability on self-assessments of health are divided into six groups, by the frequency with which a woman attends religious services, the effects of functional disability are shown to be strongest among women who never attend services. This is in contrast to the women who attend once a week or more often, whose coefficients are smaller, and almost equal. The regression slopes are graphically displayed in Figure VIII-2. The effects of disability on self-assessments of health are reduced ordinally at every level of increasing attendance at religious services, and the effects of disability at the highest levels of attendance are reduced by almost two thirds. The effects of disability on self-assessment at the highest level of religiosity even loses significance level. Thus even severely disabled women, if they are able to attend services, need not become health pessimists on the basis of their disability. The coefficient for the unmodified effect of functional disability is .125, approximately the same as that for the women who attend services every few months to once a month. But this obscures the much stronger effect of functional disability on the small group of women who never or rarely attend services. The addition of the interaction term to the model has two effects on other significant associations: it increases the coefficients for both public religiosity and income, and raises the R^2 by an almost significant increment, to .30.[2]

Standardizing the coefficients places the largest importance on the effects of the functional disability suffered by women who rarely or never attend religious services. The third largest effect is that of depression score, which was the most influential factor in the men's model. Fourth is the effect of functional disability for women who attend every few months, followed by the main effect of public religious involvement, the effect of disability on women who attend monthly, income, the effect of disability on the most frequent attenders, chronic conditions, attribution of meaning, and physical activity.

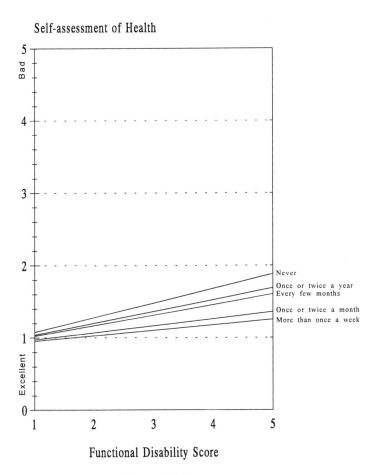

Figure VIII-2.
Effect of functional disability on women's self-assessment
of health at five levels of attendance at religious services

Summary. The *main hypothesis*, of an association between higher levels of religiosity and women's better assessments of their health, is certainly supported by the analysis. Only public, not private religious involvement, however, has this association. In addition, there are indirect and interaction effects which make the association multifaceted and complex.

The analysis fails to support the *health behavior hypothesis*; the use of alcohol is related to better assessments of health, not worse, and physical activity is again most likely acting as a health control.

The analysis also fails to support the *cohesiveness hypothesis* as explanatory of the association between religiosity and self-assessments of health, although it does clarify the relationship. That is, in contrast to the original hypothesis, women who have high levels of public religious involvement do not have more social contacts, but fewer, and since both contacts and religiosity are related to better perceptions of health, controlling for contacts enhances the association of religiosity and self-assessments of health. Thus public religiosity is related to better perceptions of health among women, not because of the larger number of social contacts among the more religiously involved, but in spite of their smaller number.

The *coherence hypothesis*, on the other hand, is supported in the expected way. Part of the reason women who are more religiously involved think they have better health is that they have stronger senses of coherence.

Finally, the *theodicy hypothesis* is also quite strongly supported by the analysis. Dividing the women into six groups by their frequency of attending religious services reveals regularly decreasing associations between functional disability and perceptions of health. The more religious participation a woman engages in, the less strongly her perceptions of health will be determined by her level of disability.

To give an idea of the magnitude of the relationships, the final model was re-estimated with interval data for the main effect of public religious involvement. Contrasting two women who are average in every way but in their religiosity, (that is, women who live in non-age-segregated housing, with medium incomes, and average activity, optimism, chronic conditions, depression, and disability levels), a woman whose religiosity is low will score 3.1 on average ("fair" health) and a woman whose religiosity is high will score 2.5 ("good-fair" health).

Discussion

One might have thought that, of all the measures of health included in this study, subjective assessments of health would be more likely to be related to religious involvement than any of the others. And while the *global hypothesis* of greater religious involvement and better perceptions of health was supported in both the men's and women's analyses, religious involvement is clearly more strongly related to women's perceptions of their health than to men's. There are no main effects of religious involvement, public or private, on men's self-assessments of health. In the men's analysis, the significant effects of public religiosity on self-assessments of health which remained when demographic factors, health behaviors, cohesiveness, and coherence had been controlled for, disappeared when objective health status entered the models. Thus, despite the theoretical expectation that religiosity would be more likely to be related to subjective, rather than objective, measures of health, public religiosity apparently has no direct effect on men's subjective evaluations of health. The hierarchical structure of the analyses, however, provides some ground for arguing that there may be an effect of religiosity that is hidden by the stringency of the methodological controls for health status. The previous analyses have shown one or the other form of religiosity to be associated with nearly all of the measures of health status. When that factor is controlled in subsequent analyses, all of the variation explained by both is subsequently treated as if it were all due to the health status measure. Whether or not there is any of this kind of "embedded" effect depends to a certain extent on the validity of the ordering of the four measures of health status. This is, ultimately, another issue of causality which can be addressed only by longitudinal research.

The first of the proposed intervening mechanisms, the *health behavior hypothesis*, receives some support, but only from the men's analysis. Men who have smoked in the past perceive their health to be poorer than men who have never smoked, and men who are more religiously-involved are less likely to smoke or to have smoked in the past. Thus some of the association between religiosity and better self-assessments of health may be attributed to the better health practices of the more religious men.

The second explanatory hypothesis, the *cohesiveness hypothesis*, produces some unexpected clarification in the women's analysis. Contrary to the prediction that women with higher levels of religious involvement would have larger numbers of social contacts, the social contact measure acts as a suppressor variable and increases, rather than decreases, the association of religiosity and perceptions of health. Thus, far from being able to attribute the more religious women's better perceptions of their health to their more numerous contacts, the interpretation must be that they have better perceptions of health in spite of their fewer contacts. There was no support for the hypothesis in the men's analysis.

Third, the *coherence hypothesis* was supported in both the men's and women's analysis. The tendency of the more religiously-involved men and women to have better self-assessments of health can be, in part, attributed to their stronger senses of coherence, indicating an important cognitive component in those subjective assessments.

The men's and women's models are alike in that, in both, it is a measure of objective health status that is most closely associated with self-assessments of health. The difference is that in the men's model it is depression that is most closely associated with self-assessments of health and in the women's model it is functional disability. This is a descriptive difference that might well be followed up in future research. Given the evidently different reference groups and criteria men and women use in assessing their health, the apparently closer association between self-assessments of health and psychological status in men, and between self-assessments of health and functional status in women may suggest something about their different definitions of health.

But recall that it was only the functional disability of the women who rarely or never attend religious services that had the strongest association--this is the second major difference. Religious participation modifies the effect of functional disability on self-assessments of health for women but not for men. And if it were not for this modifying effect, depression would be the most important factor in both analyses. This modifying effect of religious involvement is the support for the *theodicy hypothesis*, which argues that religious involvement will act to moderate the subjective perceptions of physical health problems, by giving them religious meaning. Putting them in the shared context of a theodicy relativizes the suffering, makes available a language about the experience, and a set of social relationships that one would not have otherwise. This relativizing process, in which one's own health problems are compared with others, with peers, is very much the process described in other studies as being responsible for women's better self-assessments of health when compared with men's: because women as a group have more physical and psychological health problems than do men, the self-assessments of health by individual women seem overly optimistic. Along these lines, one early study found subjects who had "high body concern," or who "expressed concern about their health" more likely to assess their health poorly (Maddox, 1962). Similarly, the finding that better self-assessments of health are also related to higher educational levels suggests that consistently different definitions of health are being employed. One major axis on which these definitions seem to turn is in the amount of emphasis or value placed on the physical self, an emphasis which might plausibly be diminished by either higher levels of education or by religious involvement. The women in this study who attended religious services more frequently had poorer functional ability for a given level of self-assessment of health, when compared with the women who attended less often or not at all. The suggestion is that religious involvement doesn't so much change definitions of health as it does alter the angle of a major hinge on which they turn.

In sum, religious involvement appears to be more strongly related to women's self-perceptions of their health than it is to men's. The retention of the main effect of religiosity and the presence of the interaction effect indicate that religious involvement explains some of the variation in women's self-perceptions of health that cannot be accounted for in any other way proposed here. Moreover, it is the social aspects of religious involvement which are related, not the private aspects, even in the interaction. Thus a very basic perception that these women have about themselves appears to be influenced, in more than one way, by their social participation in religious activities.

Subjective perceptions of health are evidently extremely sensitive to an apparently fundamental, underlying sense of an individual's well-being. The mechanisms by which this highly tuned level of consciousness operates are unknown. But the combination of the question's elegant economy and the power of its prediction in longitudinal studies make its continued use in survey research a virtual certainty. At the same time, the range of factors associated with self-assessment of health, here and in other research, suggests that a very complex structure of meanings of health and illness is being elicited. It is a structure which is tied to an individual's objective social location, but it produces criteria which are consciously, subjectively, evaluated. The perceptiveness of the process is manifested in its correlation with longevity, which demonstrates the salience of the element of consciousness in affecting objective health levels. What the present analysis demonstrates is the ability of social factors to modify those perceptions.

Notes for Chapter VIII

[1] The equation for the final model is written:

$$Y = 1.37 + .05X_{1a} - .03X_{1b} - .10X_2 + .09X_3 -$$

$$.03X_4 + .07X_5 + .11X_6 + .03X_7$$

Where X_{1a} = Public v. "other" housing
X_{1b} = Private v. "other" housing
X_2 = Public religiosity index
X_3 = Private religiosity index
X_4 = Physical activity index
X_5 = Chronic conditions index
X_6 = Functional disability index
X_7 = Depression index

[2] The equation for the final model can be written:

$$Y = .876 + .75X_{1a} + .09X_{1b} - .31X_2 - .02X_3$$

$$+ .19X_{4a} + .17X_{4b} - .02X_5 - .04X_6 + .09X_7$$

$$+ .03X_8 + .20X_{9a} + .16X_{9b} + .10X_{9d}$$

$$+ .07X_{9e} + .07X_{9f}$$

Where X_{1a} = Public v. "other" housing
X_{1b} = Private v. "other" housing
X_2 = Public religiosity index
X_3 = Private religiosity index
X_{4a} = High v. low income
X_{4b} = Medium v. low income
X_5 = Physical activity index
X_6 = Meaning index
X_7 = Chronic conditions index
X_8 = Depression index
X_{9a} = Functional disability / Never attends
X_{9b} = Functional disability / Once or twice a year

X_{9c} = Functional disability / Every few months
X_{9d} = Functional disability / Once or twice a month
X_{9e} = Functional disability / Once a week
X_{9f} = Functional disability / More than once a week

Plotting the predicted values for the final model against the residual values shows no evidence of heteroscedasticity. The model appears to predict slightly better for women with numerous chronic illnesses, but in general the residuals are randomly distributed.

IX
Religious Bodies

The analysis has demonstrated the existence of a multi-faceted association between religious involvement and the health of a sample of New Haven elderly. The association is a uniformly positive one; greater religious involvement is associated with lower levels of chronic conditions, better functional ability, more optimistic self-perceptions of health, and less depression. Many qualifications of this statement need to be made, however; the purpose of the discussion must be to spell out both the implications of the analysis and its limitations. Beginning with the fundamental circumscription that this is a cross-sectional study, the analysis has two heavy obligations: to be as widely exploratory, and as internally structured as possible. Only by considering the widest range of plausible explanatory mechanisms, and by fixing certain stationary points from which to make comparative assessments, can one effectively do what cross-sectional studies are intended to do, and that is to describe the patterns in the data.

In this final chapter, the minutiae of the analyses will be summarized from the general theoretical perspectives of Chapters I and II. The findings will be contrasted and compared using the two structural elements built into the analyses: the separate analyses for men and women, and the cumulative health controls. It has been the goal of this highly interdisciplinary investigation to place religious involvement in the context of the debate over the role of psychosocial factors in health. The intent of Chapters I and II was to use the specific perspective of classical sociological theories of religion to develop a theoretical framework in which the diverse forms of religious involvement might plausibly have effects on human health. Four explanatory mechanisms were proposed; three (the health behavior, cohesiveness, and coherence hypotheses) that treated religious involvement as a main effect, and one (the theodicy hypothesis) that proposed that the relevance of religious involvement to health would be limited to situations of specific stress. The arguments were developed to analogously coincide with the two sides of the predominant debate over psychosocial factors in health: that social support is important in health either because it interacts with stresses in the environment, or, alternatively, because it has main effects of its own. Sidney Cobb has argued recently that the distinction between main effects and interaction effects is "not worth worrying about," for two reasons. First, he says, few lives are without social or psychological stress, so the interaction with stress at the lowest levels simply looks like a main effect. By the same token, few lives are totally isolated, so that at the very lowest levels of social support, the deprivation would become a stress in itself (Cobb, 1979). Perhaps at this level of generality, where there is no zero point on the scale, the two kinds of effects cannot be distinguished. When dealing with more specific manifestations of psychosocial factors, however, such as religious involvement, which can be totally absent, or present to a greater or lesser degree, the question of main versus interactive effects becomes concrete and open to testing and interpretation. The description of main effects, moreover, can be enhanced by the introduction of intervening explanatory mechanisms; the description of interactions by the use of concrete and specific measures of stress and support. Thus the test of these ideas with specific forms of religious involvement and stress concretely operationalized in the form of objective measures of illness, is only a limited test of these broad issues. Only with an accretion of such limited tests, however, is the matter likely to be resolved.

Assessing the Hypotheses: I

The theoretical perspective outlined in Chapter I made a main effects argument, that religious involvement would be directly related to better health, and that it might be related indirectly through the mechanisms of health behaviors, social cohesiveness, or cognitive coherence. As it turns out, there are both direct and indirect effects evident in the data. Table IX-1. summarizes the associations found in the men's and women's analyses of the four health measures. Let us first summarize the evidence for the three hypotheses, that health behaviors, social cohesiveness, or a sense of coherence in some way account for the relationship of religious involvement and health.

The Health Behavior Hypothesis. Behaviorialist approaches in the social sciences explicitly do not consider beliefs or experiences as matters for study. In that sense then, the behavioral hypothesis for the present study may be considered mis-named, because it is based on actions undertaken on the basis of specific contents of religious belief, not on reflexive behaviors. But in fact it is appropriate, because no argument is being made that the belief in the health benefit of the religious/health practice is required; the health practices in question are factors with demonstrated physiological-causal relationships to morbidity and/or mortality, and knowledge of their health benefit need not be a condition of their efficacy. The health behaviors have direct effects of their own in many of the analyses, particularly in the analysis of the chronic conditions index, in which there were direct, positive associations of chronic conditions with smoking, being overweight and physically inactive. All of these three were somewhat associated, in the independent variable analysis in Chapter IV, with attending religious services and knowing many in one's congregation, but only physical activity consistently reduced the association between public religiosity and health. It did this in the analysis of every single health measure that had a first-order correlation with public religiosity (that is, seven out of the eight analyses). The interpretation given has been that physical activity is acting straightforwardly as a health control, and since its effects are usually reduced by the addition of subsequent health controls, this must be at least partly correct.

Table IX-1. Summary of significant effects

	Chronic Conditions	Functional Disability	Depression	Self-Assessment of Health
MAIN EFFECTS				
Public	<	< >	<	<
Private				
Health Behavior		<		>
INDIRECT EFFECTS				
Cohesiveness			>	
Coherence				< >
INTERACTIONS				
Public				<
Private		>	>	

< = women;   > = men

As Table IX-1. shows, however, in two of the analyses there are significant associations of the health measures with health practices other than physical activity, associations which do reduce the association between public religiosity and health. These two instances are in the analysis of women's functional disability, in which the combined effects of never having smoked, not being overweight, and engaging in more physical activity, accounted for more than a quarter of the association between public religiosity and better functional ability; and in the analysis of men's self-assessments of health, where the combination of never having smoked, and being physically active accounts for more than a third of the tendency for more publicly religious men to have better self-assessments of health. Thus there is some support for the explanatory mechanism of the behavioral hypothesis; there is some evidence to suggest that the better health practices of the religiously-involved, particularly their disinclination to smoke, in part accounts for their better health. Moreover, the strength and consistent positive directions of the associations between the various health practices and the specific forms of religious involvement reported in Chapter IV suggest several new lines of investigation. The behavioral hypothesis should certainly be included in future longitudinal studies of religious involvement and health, and religious involvement should also be included in studies of the determinants of health behaviors.

The Social Cohesiveness Hypothesis. As tests of the social cohesiveness hypothesis, the social network variables yield fewer results to discuss. There is only one indirect effect of public or private religiosity through some social network factor, and that was in the analysis of men's depression, as Table IX-1. shows. Men who attended religious services more frequently were less depressed on average, but married men were far more likely to attend services than were the formerly married, and when marital status was controlled, the relationship between religious involvement and depression disappeared. With this single exception then, it appears that no part of the relationship between religious involvement and better health can be attributed to the fact that the religiously-involved have larger or more intimate social networks than the non-religiously-involved. As was the case with the health behaviors, though, there are numerous associations with individual network measures which should attract further analysis.

The more surprising result may be that there are no main effects of the social network measures on their own. It should be remembered, however, that the major studies showing the effects of social network measures in health have been longitudinal studies of mortality rates. There is no basis for extrapolating from them to morbidity studies, certainly not to studies of morbidity among the elderly, where survivor effects greatly complicate the matter. Indeed, the recent study by Stoller (1984) showed that it was the elderly with the *most* functional impairment who received the most informal social assistance. If social support is positively related to disability and negatively related to mortality, there is the potential for finding a suppression effect with a mortality outcome, but it also underscores the complexity of the social support measure, disclosing a new form of constraint it imposes those who receive its benefits: feelings of dependency and helplessness. Indeed, the only other significant association of a social network measure, besides the impact of men's marital status on depression, was the small effect of social contact on women's self-assessments of health, and that disappeared when fatalism was controlled at the next step. To complicate matters somewhat, but perhaps to clarify them, there was some evidence in the analysis of women's self-assessments of health that publicly-religious women had better assessments of their health, not because of their larger numbers of social contacts, but in spite of their smaller numbers. If elderly women who are relatively isolated successfully find social companionship through their religious activities, that compensation would be invisible in this analysis. The conclusion one must draw is that the relationship of religious involvement and social networks is too complex to be described by these crude measures, and that more descriptive studies should be undertaken.

The Coherence Hypothesis. In connection with the coherence hypothesis, a widely-read recent social scientific theory of religion (Greeley, 1982) argues that religious feelings and beliefs originate in the individual's propensity to hope, and that the more of this propensity they possess, the more religious they will be. While the present analysis cannot address the weighty problem of the origins of religious belief, it does provide a way of seeing if hopefulness and religious involvement are coterminous, and also if they have similar associations with health. As a construct, the attribution of meaning was positively related to *all* of the forms of religious involvement; the attribution of fatalism was not related to any.

The test of the coherence hypothesis is different from the previous two in that the measures of meaning and fatalism tend to be rather strongly associated with many of the health measures, having main effects of their own. At the same time, it is similar in that there are just a few indirect effects of religious involvement through the sense of coherence. As Table IX-1. shows, the only indirect effects are in the analyses of both men's and women's self-assessments of health; in both, public (not private) religiosity has an indirect positive association with subjective assessments of health through the sense of coherence. That is, publicly religiously-involved individuals tend to have better self-assessments of health partly because they also have a stronger sense of coherence. But these associations are fairly small, accounting for just over 10 percent of the religiosity-self-assessment relationship in the women's model and just over 20 percent in the men's.

Thus the sense of coherence, at least as it is presently operationalized, is not a sufficient explanatory mechanism for understanding the total association between religious involvement and health. If a sense of coherence has any intervening role at all, it is limited to accounting for some effects of public religiosity only. Importantly, however, the attributions of meaning and fatalism have substantial associations of their own with most of the health measures. Either or both are directly or indirectly associated with the health measure in every analysis except that of women's chronic conditions. They play their most important roles in the analyses of depression, where the attribution of meaning is the single most important factor associated with both men's and women's depression. In the analysis, meaning and fatalism even carry an interaction of their own, suggesting that the combination of high levels of meaninglessness and fatalism presents a situation of especially high risk of depression. With regard to the other measures of health, fatalism and meaning are related to subjective assessments of health both directly, and indirectly through the more objective health measures. These constructs of meaning and fatalism are evidently highly sensitive to the perceptions and expressions of health among this group of elderly people, and show great potential utility for further research.

The Main Hypothesis. The main effects of public and private religiosity, left when all hypotheses and health controls have been considered, are in some ways the most mysterious of the associations. They are the residual associations remaining when the effects of all available explanatory mechanisms are accounted for, found in the lefthand column of Table IX-1. Such direct relationships between religious involvement and health are evident for all measures of health. Public religiosity is directly and positively related to fewer chronic conditions, lower functional disability and depression and to better self-assessments of health among women, and to lower functional disability among men. Private religiosity holds no main effect relationships with any health measure; its only significant first-order correlation with any health measure was in the analysis of men's depression, an association which disappeared when one form of private religiosity appeared in an interaction. The meaning of these associations depends completely on some set of intervening mechanisms that is apparently different from those tested here. The fact that only public religious activities are involved is suggestive.

It raises the very Durkheimian view that religious feelings originate in collective rites. Are there some very basic, even physiological characteristics that pertain to the shared experience of religious services and rituals? At what they call the "biogenetic structural" level of analysis, d'Aquili et al. (1979) propose that ritual, religious ritual most especially, produces a unique physiological experience which coordinates and synchronizes the brain and the body. More popular theories along this line have included Benson's (1984) *Beyond the Relaxation Response*, where he argues that the "faith factor" activated by meditation or prayer, enhances health by reducing stress. Such a direct physiological effect of religious experience would be a plausible way of explaining the residual main effects of public religiosity, but it is not the only way. Moreover, to the extent that such an explanation ignores the symbolic content of religious experience, it can fairly be accused of simplistic reductionism. Turning this process on its head, psychologists going back to William James have observed that religious interpretations are frequently given to states of physiological and emotional arousal (James, 1978 [1901-1902]; Sargant, 1969; Proudfoot and Shaver, 1975). The implication of all of these studies is that the physiological component and its conscious interpretation in the religious experience deserve much further study.

Assessing the Hypotheses: II

The consideration of the importance of the physiological elements in the Chapter I association of religious involvement and health, leads us into the Chapter II argument, that an interactive effect is involved. If states of physiological and emotional arousal are more likely than non-aroused states to be given religious interpretation, then conditions of physical illness and suffering would be especially likely to be the object of such cognitions.

The significance of and concern for human suffering has been a major, continuous theme in the major Western religious traditions. Physical, bodily pain carries great meaning. The pre-eminent symbol of Christianity is the crucifixion and its ennobling of suffering. And while Judaic interpretations of the causes of suffering have tended to appeal more to history than to personal circumstance, some of the most expressive and specific religious writing on illness and suffering appears in the books of Job and the Psalms.

The specific content of these theodicies of bodily suffering, of course, cannot be addressed by the data. The point simply is that numerous interpretive schemes, some of which were indicated in Chapter II, are available in the Judeo-Christian tradition. The contribution the present analysis makes to a further study of such theodicies in particular and the interactive effects of religious involvement as an example of psychosocial factors in health in general is that the interactions in the data are highly specific, in regard both to the stresses involved (illnesses) and the form of religious involvement. The conclusion reached in Chapter I, that interaction effects are most likely to be found when the measures of both stress and support are quite specific, seems to have been supported.

Overall, there are three significant interactions in the analyses in which a specific form of religious involvement modifies the effects of a more objective measure of health on a more subjective measure of health. Specifically, a man's feeling that he receives a great deal of strength and comfort from religion reduces the effects of chronic conditions on the level of disability he suffers. Also, a man's feelings of religious identity mitigate the effects of disability on depression. For women, on the other hand, it is a form of public religious involvement that plays this modifying role: across six levels of frequency of attendance at religious services, at every greater level of attendance the tendency of disability to produce poor self-assessments of health is reduced. The two interactions with disability suggest that subjective feelings of depression or evaluations of the state of one's health will be less strictly determined by one's physical state if one carries a religious interpretation of them than if one does not.

The first observation which should be made about these three interactions is that the standardized coefficient for the effects of disability or chronic conditions at the level of never attending religious services, receiving no comfort at all from religion, or perceiving oneself to be not at all religious, is the largest, or one of the largest coefficients in the model. This happens because religious involvement tends to interact with the most important factors in each analysis, with the result that it places the individuals in the least religious category at or near the greatest risk of functional disability, depression, or poor assessment of health.

The significance of these interactions echoes the finding of the Zuckerman, Kasl, and Ostfeld (1984) study which found an interactive effect between religiousness and morbidity in predicting follow-up mortality rates. In that study the indication of the private religious feeling of getting comfort from religion was more strongly protective against mortality among the elderly than was the public involvement of church attendance. The significant interaction disclosed that among the elderly in good health, religiousness was *not* predictive of mortality. They concluded that the role of religiousness was apparently not in preventing new episodes of morbidity, but in preventing serious episodes from becoming fatal ones. We conclude that religiousness may also play a role in preventing chronic physical illness and its disabling effects from becoming demoralizing.

One of the major boundaries circumscribing the discussion is that all interpretations of the results must be considered specific to the elderly. One might speculate that the interaction effects between illness and religiousness are especially likely to be age-specific, given the prevalence of chronic illness among the elderly. There was some evidence in Chapter IV that, while the elderly as a group were quite strongly religious, the very oldest New Haven elderly were most likely to be strongly privately religious. Given the role that private religious involvement seems to play in moderating the effects of physical illness on disability, and disability on depression, the interactions become perhaps more predictable among the elderly, but also more substantively significant.

But there is another reason these findings may be particular to the elderly, a reason that has more to do with the content of religious beliefs than with their functions. As a body of beliefs and knowledge, religion is permanent, traditional. It can be accumulated over the life span at the same time that it is deepened by personal experience. The development of religiousness over the life course is a perspective that is commonly assumed (Vaux, 1984), but is now also the basis for an extensive psychological theory of the development of faith (Fowler, 1981). The Judeo-Christian tradition, on the whole, has had a tradition of respect for the aged, manifested most clearly in the numerous institutions and social welfare services sponsored by churches and synagogues. The implication of all of this is that, while the best place to look for relationships between religion and health, may be among the elderly, it may also be the only place they are found, and generalizations to other age groups must not be made unless other evidence is available.

Just as important as the outside boundary circumscribing the interpretation of the results, is an internal dividing line, the differences between men and women. The structure of separate-sex analyses becomes a kind of Archimedean point from which to view these relationships. Given the large data set, the exploratory nature of the analysis, and the expected differences between men and women in regard to both health and religious involvement, the separate-sex analyses are an asset for a cross-sectional study. If the results are the same for the two sexes, that would be a kind of internal replication. If they are different, the question must be, do they make sense according to what else is known about sex differences?

The outcome is that there are substantial differences between the men and women in the study, and they do tend to fall into a pattern. There are both quantitative and qualitative differences. First, there is some main or interactive association of religion with every single one of the health measures analyzed, for women. Religion fails to appear in one of the men's analyses, that of chronic conditions. For women both the main and interactive effects are of *public*, not private religiosity. Recall the importance of the participatory, social, public religiosity in the women's log linear analysis of religiosity, networks, and sense of coherence. Attending religious services and knowing many people in her congregation are the determining features of a woman's religious involvement and sense of coherence. They are the most characteristic attributes, the most revealing aspects of the total pattern of relationships. Recall also that this can be in part explained by the fact that a large number of the women are widowed and widowed women are especially likely to attend religious services frequently. Widowed men, on the other hand, are more likely than married men to *never* attend services. The consequences of these sex differences for the health analyses are most clearly demonstrated in the analysis of men's depression scores. In that analysis, when marital status was controlled, the previously-existing relationship between public religiosity and depression disappeared: men who attended services more were less depressed because they were more likely to be married. There would seem to be some influence here, of married women on their husbands, to attend religious services more frequently; when bereaved, women increase their attendance and men decrease theirs.

The women are more fatalistic than the men; that is, they express more helplessness, fewer feelings of personal control. But at the same time they are no less hopeful than men are, no less able to find meaning in their present situation and hope for the future. This is linked to women's greater overall religiosity: in the log linear analysis, women who knew many other people in their congregation were most likely to be both *hopeful* and *helpless*, that is, subject to feelings of fatalism but maintaining a strong sense that life is meaningful. This certainly suggests that elderly women in difficult circumstances seek comfort in the social life of the church or temple congregation, and while this may not diminish their feelings of helplessness or enhance their sense of control, it does give them hope. This sense of meaningfulness is no less important in its association with depression in men, the difference being that for men it is not in any way mediated through religion. Instead, it is to be found in an interaction with fatalism, indicating the sensitivity of men's feelings of depression to the combination of extreme helplessness and hopelessness.

It does appear that the public, social aspects of religious involvement have a more salient association with women's health than with men's, judging from the main effects of public religiosity in every measure of women's health, and that the only significant interaction found for women included a form of public religiosity. I have tried to put this as neutrally as possible, because there are two rather different ways of interpreting this, depending on which causal directions are involved. The first is that the ubiquity of both public and private religious involvement among elderly women may actually be producing its own ill health, in a way, by making deviants of non-religious women. This would be more relevant to women than to men because elderly women are more religiously involved overall, and because the behavioral manifestations in public involvement are more readily observable. The other possibility is that women simply do suffer more than men do from the objective conditions of chronic illness and bereavement, and tend to seek out religious comfort to fill their greater needs.

The finding of sex-specific patterns in the relationship of religious involvement and health suggests that the finding in the House, Robbins, and Metzner (1982) study, that only church attendance, alone among the types of social relationships examined, was significantly related to women's mortality rates. The present study suggests that this may not be an anomalous finding, but the predictable result of the fact that the only form of religious involvement they asked about was attendance at services. The present finding, of quantitatively greater and qualitatively different religious involvement for women, and the stronger association with health, contributes to the understanding of sex differences in both religious involvement and in health.

Conscious Deindividuation

There is an overarching construct available for characterizing the overall effect of religion in health, if indeed, further evidence of one is demonstrated. The concept of conscious deindividuation combines the elements of the ideas of cohesiveness and coherence that are relevant to religious belief and practice, and integrates them. The term deindividuation is used here as it is used in psychological research, to designate a highly specific state in which an individual's surroundings make it difficult for him to discriminate himself from others. It has been used to describe situations in which individuals have little awareness of their uniqueness, in groups in which members have few distinctions between them. The concept of deindividuation is considered a cultural variant in the determination of objective self-awareness, the condition of focusing attention on oneself (Wicklund, 1975).

Wicklund's work and review of related studies shows that attention is basically dichotomous; it can be focused inwardly and take the self as an object, or it can be directed outwardly, to some feature of the environment. Research on the condition of objective self-awareness consistently finds that, when individuals are forced to focus on themselves, (by having to sit in front of a mirror, or hearing tape recordings of their own voice), they tend to appraise themselves more negatively than individuals who are not provoked to self-awareness. Thus, distractions which pull attention away from the self, or cultures which do not promote expressions of individual uniqueness, will protect individuals from the negative evaluations of themselves caused by self-scrutiny. When individual thought-processes merge imperceptibly into the group's thought processes, the inner life becomes indistinguishable from the shared life. At the other extreme, isolated individuals may become elaborately introspective.

The negative evaluations produced by objective self-awareness were found to result in measurable levels of psychological distress in a study recently reported by Mechanic (1979). In a 16-year follow-up of 302 young adults who had been studied when they were children, Mechanic found that introspectiveness, indicated by the individual's responses that they were "sensitive and introspective," "worried about meaning in life," and "interested in psychology," was more highly correlated with psychological distress than any other factor. Mechanic uses Jerome Frank's term "demoralization" to characterize what he means by psychological distress, ". . . a learned pattern of illness behavior involving an intense focus on internal feeling states, careful monitoring of body sensations, and a high level of self-awareness" (1979, p. 1234).

There is a reflexive relation here between self-attention and the experience of distress or pain. Pain is individuating, in that it draws the individual's attention away from the environment, toward itself. At the same time, actions that direct individuals' attention toward themselves increase the perception of pain. In a very suggestive clinical study of the use of language by elderly women patients with depression, Bucci and Freedman (1981) noted the apparent inability of their subjects to take the point of view of another person, even the person to whom they were talking. Their patients' five-minute monologues (on whatever they wanted to talk about) contained many more first person singular pronouns than did the monologues of a group of normal subjects. The women patients were also very low in referential activity, rarely referring to objects in the environment or to concrete events. Instead, their conversations focused entirely on their subjective reactions to things, and were "rambling, repetitious and vague" (p. 348). As the clinical status of these women improved, they began to use more second and third person pronouns, and became more colorful and descriptive in their accounts, but also more expressive of their suffering. Bucci and Freedman marked the beginning of their patients' clinical improvement with their recognition and verbal description of their distress. The implication is that the language used to communicate the distress depends on a minimal level of intersubjective awareness, an individual's ability to extend attention beyond themselves.

The construct of conscious deindividuation describes the hypothesized social and cognitive effects of religion in health. By itself, the term deindividuation characterizes simply the integrating and regulating, the belonging and constraining functions of religion, the Durkheimian view we have called cohesiveness. The modifier "conscious" is appended to give it the intentional character of the cognitive activity of giving religious meaning to events and feelings. The measures of private religiosity in the survey are indications of an experiential, conscious aspect of religion. They are acknowledgements of the individual's self-attention or introspection given a religious interpretation. They are indications that the individual has engaged in religious reflectiveness to the extent that they think of themselves as being religious people.

They are also evidently indications of the efficacy of that experience in situations of need, insofar as so many of the respondents felt that they received "a great deal of strength and comfort from religion." The description of this process as a conscious one is supported by the interactions of the measures of religiosity with helplessness and disability. In situations of objective, physical helplessness, the deliberate, intentional merging of the self with the wider religious group renders the situation less hopeless, and is reflected in less disability and depression, and more optimistic subjective perceptions of health. A similar dynamic was observed by Andreasen and Norris in their study of burn patients: "Most patients resolve this identity crisis by using a fairly consistent set of adaptive mechanisms that help them redefine their sense of identity on a nonphysical foundation, using increased family ties, greater emphasis on inner worth, religiosity, etc." (1972, p. 352).

Another close description of the construct is to be found in William James' *The Varieties of Religious Experience*:

> . . . the man identifies his real being with the germinal higher part of himself; and does so in the following way. *He becomes conscious that this higher part is conterminous and continuous with a MORE of the same quality, which is operative in the universe outside of him, and which he can keep in working touch with, and in a fashion get on board of and save himself when all his lower being has gone to pieces in the wreck.*
>
> . . . confining ourselves to what is common and generic, we have in *the fact that the conscious person is continuous with a wider self through which saving experiences come*, a positive content of religious experience which, it seems to me, is literally and objectively true as far as it goes. (1978 [1901-1902] pp. 489, 495, his emphases).

It can also be found in Gordon Allport's description of the symbol of the cross as "'the I, crossed out'"; "What is demanded by the great religions is self-abnegation, discipline, surrender. To find one's life one must lose it" (1950, pp. 29, 22). The construct of conscious deindividuation attempts to capture the essence of this religious impulse, to describe deliberate, religiously-motivated selflessness, and to find in that element of religious experience, which, as James wrote, "is true as far as it goes" the source of hope in the context of helplessness.

The Body is the Metaphor: Classical Sociological Theory and Epidemiology

This study had twin goals: in addition to the concrete empirical evaluation of some epidemiological evidence on the relationship of religious involvement and the health of the elderly, it has sought to demonstrate the wealth of insight the classical sociological tradition has to offer the contemporary enterprise of social epidemiology. The time has come to be specific about what that contribution is.

Any question about social factors in health is an inherently functional one. Epidemiology is the study of the distribution of disease throughout the group as a whole. The concept of a prevalence rate, for example, is very precise, but totally abstract; it does not in any way refer to individuals. The concept of an individual's relative risk, by comparison, is very crude, except for those diseases that have easily-measured environmental causes, and that have been studied a great deal. In epidemiology, the individual can only be comprehended as a member of one or more groups. Prevalence rates refer to *social* groups. These are groups whose boundaries are specified, and which usually have some common-sense referent by virtue of their coinciding with political, geographic, or other boundaries. So a prevalence rate is a condition of a social whole, an indicator of the health of the social totality. This is precisely the kind of evidence Durkheim was analyzing in *Suicide*, and from which he drew the conclusion that society was a reality *sui generis*, and that its suicide rate was "an echo of the moral state . . . of the whole social body" (1951 [1897], p. 300).

What Durkheimian social theory and epidemiology have in common is a metaphor. The title of this chapter, "Religious Bodies" is a deliberate play on words, intended to blur the distinction between the human body and the body of believers. The ambiguity is hardly a novel observation on my part; the use of the metaphor of the physical body of Christ to refer to the Christian church dates from the earliest recorded writings. Describing a social group by likening it to the body is by no means limited to religious groups, however, using the body as a metaphor is universal and fundamental to systems of cognition (Hertz, 1960 [1907]; Douglas, 1973). In a fascinating discussion of the use of metaphor in everyday language, Lakoff and Johnson (1980) call the body a "basic domain of experience," "an experiential gestalt." The physical environment and the social environment are the two other fundamentally "natural kinds of experience" (p. 117). These are the most concrete kinds of experience, the most physical and least cultural we can have. The body structures concepts at many levels of abstraction, beginning with some as primary as being and non-being, or inside and outside. Bodies are the location for the center of spatial organization, and they are the *a priori* object, an entity bounded by a surface. Further, they are made up of sets of parts that are related in certain typical ways making up a characteristic, but largely hidden, structure.

The body has also been a highly useful metaphor for modern social science, beginning with Durkheim's *The Division of Labor in Society*. Generations of undergraduate sociology students have been confused by the apparently illogical names Durkheim applied to the earlier and later stages of society, mechanical and organic solidarity. This probably says more about the pervasiveness of the value placed on technology in our society than it does about Durkheim, but unless one thinks about these names as metaphors, they really do not seem to make sense. Bodies are produced by nature, we reason, but it takes culture to make a machine. As metaphors for the relationships of parts to wholes, however, they make a lot of sense.

Mechanical solidarity is what holds primitive, or in Durkheim's scheme, "segmental" societies together, the "solidarity which comes from likenesses," (1964 [1893], p. 130). "The social molecules" act together "as the molecules of organic bodies" (p. 130). Mechanical solidarity is a much weaker form of social cohesion than the organic solidarity which develops out of it. The metaphor of the machine, then, gives way to the metaphor of the body. Durkheim not only gives this process graphic precision by using the metaphor of cell division and differentiation to describe the transition, but the metaphor decides the final concept: modern, complex social bodies are made up of organs and organ systems. Cell division is the metaphorical source of change: population growth, which results in the intensification of social life, is the engine that runs the division of labor. Competition produces diversity and specialization.

Organic solidarity, then, is the condition of societies in which people are bound together by their differences, which are systematically organized into a division of labor. Durkheim marshalls the power of heterosexual attraction as support for his theory that the solidarity between opposites is stronger than the solidarity between similars, and that even the sexual division of labor has been increasing. Moreover, Durkheim invests this social life principle with moral significance. Because organic solidarity requires mutual dependence, anti-social activities such as crime are also immoral because they weaken the whole structure. Tellingly, Durkheim uses the body metaphor to illuminate the crucial concept of social deviance, likening it to infection (p. 224), cancer, or tuberculosis (p. 353). The social system is the tissue through which social events penetrate, and those which serve to break it down are pathological.

The epidemiological perspective is inevitably a functionalist one. And while epidemiologists may be interested in morbidity and mortality for their own sakes, sociologists can treat this information as illuminative of social structures and processes. In fact, this research ends up being strong support for functionalism, Durkheimian functionalism, at that. This is another form of pathology that defines normality. The association of religious involvement with better health cannot be described as simply a latent function of religion, not when the processes are as evidently conscious as the interactions depict them to be. There is an important distinction to be made between the function of religion for the individual and the function of religion for society. The link between them is epidemiological--if religion benefits individual health then it does function for society through individuals.

The best part of Durkheim's use of metaphor, however, is his willingness to carry it all the way to its meaningful conclusion. Society for him was analogous to an organism not just in its structure; it had self-consciousness, or *conscience* as well. Just as the brain expresses and completes the unity of the organism, so the whole of society "takes conscience" of itself. In fact, Durkheim argues that collective self-consciousness is both prior to and necessary for the development of individual self-consciousness. The human self-consciousness contained within the body is thus the crucial element in the metaphor for describing the role religion played in Durkheim's thought. It was precisely in the religious life that social self-consciousness, from which individual self-consciousness is derived, appears.

In the present analysis, great stress has been laid on the consciously *sought-for* nature of private religious involvement, and this argues against any characterization based on latent functionality. The apparent relevance of religious involvement to situations of objective suffering confirms the Weberian view that religion implies a constitution of meaning, a self-determined choice of interpretation. Thus the cohesiveness and the coherence of the social group are, in a sense, writ small in the individual, but in a way over which he or she has some control.

The relevance of both Durkheimian and Weberian sociological theories of religion to contemporary social epidemiology is thus demonstrated. Both of these major theoretical perspectives contribute to the interpretation of the data; the concept of conscious deindividuation is an attempt to distill the relevance of each to each other, in a way that makes them both relevant to health. This analysis underscores the critical importance of psychosocial factors in health in two ways. In finding evidence for a complex direct and interactive association between religion and health, it opens up an area of research which is theoretically rich and carries the potential for clarifying many of the issues pertaining to social factors in general.

It also provides much evidence along the way for the influence of the subjective reality in health. There is an element of consciousness in health that is not purely determined by the individual's physical status. The classical theory traditions yield a broad foundation on which to build an understanding of the operative mechanisms in the association between religious involvement and health, within which there is plenty of room for contemporary ingenuity. What they do not leave in doubt is the prediction that the association will be a positive one.

Bibliography

Abramson, Lyn Y., Martin E. P. Seligman, and John D. Teasdale. "Learned Helplessness in Humans: Critique and Reformulation." *Journal of Abnormal Psychology* 87(1978):49-74.

Achenbaum, W. Andrew. *Old Age in the New Land*. Baltimore: Johns Hopkins University Press, 1978.

Allport, Gordon W. *The Individual and His Religion: A Psychological Interpretation*. New York: MacMillan Company, 1950.

Alston, Jon P. and William Alex McIntosh. "An Assessment of the Determinants of Religious Participation." *Sociological Quarterly* 20(1979):49-62.

American Public Health Association. *Health of Minorities and Women*. Washington, D.C.: American Public Health Association, 1982.

Andreasen, N.J.C. and A.S. Norris. "Long-Term Adjustment and Adaptation Mechanisms in Severely Burned Adults." *The Journal of Nervous and Mental Disease* 154(1972):352-362.

Antonovsky, Aaron. *Health, Stress, and Coping*. San Francisco: Jossey-Bass, Inc., 1980.

d'Aquili, Eugene G., Charles D. Laughlin, and John McManus. *The Spectrum of Ritual: A Biogenetic Structural Analysis*. New York: Columbia University Press, 1979.

Argyle, Michael. *Religious Behavior*. London: Routledge & Kegan Paul, 1958.

Aron, Raymond. *Main Currents in Sociological Thought II: Durkheim/Pareto/Weber*. Translated by Richard Howard and Helen Weaver. New York: Basic Books, 1967.

Ayuso-Gutierrez, J.L., F.Fuentenebro de Diego, and I. Mateo Martin. "Psychosocial Factors in Later Life Depression." *International Journal of Social Psychiatry* 28(1982):137-140.

Bahr, Howard M. "Aging and Religious Disaffiliation." *Social Forces* 49(1970):59-71.

Bakan, David. *Disease, Pain and Sacrifice: Toward a Psychology of Suffering*. Boston: Beacon Press, 1968.

Barnes, J.A. "Social Networks." Addison-Wesley Modular Publications, No. 26, 1972.

Bartlett, F.C. *Remembering: A Study in Experimental and Social Psychology*. London: Cambridge University Press, 1932.

Beck, Aaron T. *Depression: Causes and Treatment*. Philadelphia: University of Pennsylvania Press, 1967.

Becker, Ernest. *The Denial of Death*. New York: Free Press, 1973.

Bellah, Robert. *Beyond Belief: Essays on Religion in a Post-Traditional World*. New York: Harper & Row, 1970.

Benson, Herbert. *Beyond the Relaxation Response*. New York: New York Times Books, 1984.

Berger, Peter L. *The Sacred Canopy: Elements of a Sociological Theory of Religion*. New York: Doubleday, 1967.

Berger, Peter L. and Thomas Luckmann. *The Social Construction of Reality: A Treatise in the Sociology of Knowledge*. New York: Doubleday, 1967.

Berkman, Lisa F. and S. Leonard Syme. "Social Networks, Host Resistance, and Mortality: A Nine-Year Follow-Up Study of Alameda County Residents." *American Journal of Epidemiology* 115(1979):186-204.

Blazer, Dan G. "Social Support and Mortality in an Elderly Community Population." *American Journal of Epidemiology* 115(1982):684-694.

Blazer, Dan G. and Erdman Palmore. "Religion and Aging in a Longitudinal Panel." *The Gerontologist* Vol.16 No.1 Pt.1(1976):82-85.

Boissevain, Jeremy and J. Clyde Mitchell, editors. *Network Analysis: Studies in Human Interaction.* The Hague: Mouton, 1973.

Bott, Elizabeth. *Family and Social Network.* London: Tavistock, 1957.

Bowker, John. *Problems of Suffering in the Religions of the World.* Cambridge: Cambridge University Press, 1970.

Bowker, John. *The Sense of God: Sociological, Anthropological, and Psychological Approaches to the Origin of the Sense of God.* Oxford: Clarendon Press, 1973.

Bowlby, John. *Attachment.* 2nd edition. New York: Basic Books, 1969.

Brigham, Amariah. *Observations on the Influence of Religion Upon the Health and Physical Welfare of Mankind.* Boston: Marsh, Capen & Lyon, 1835 (New York: Arno Press, 1973).

Broverman, Inge, Susan Vogel, Donald Broverman, Frank Clarkson, and Paul Rosenkrantz. "Sex-Role Stereotypes: A Current Appraisal." *Journal of Social Issues* 28(1972):59-78.

Brown, George W. and Tirril Harris. *Social Origins of Depression: A Study of Psychiatric Disorder in Women.* London: Tavistock, 1978.

Bucci, Wilma and Norbert Freedman. "The Language of Depression."
Bulletin of the Menninger Clinic 45(1981):334-358.

Bulman, Ronnie Janoff and Camille Wortman. "Attributions of Blame
and Coping in the 'Real World': Severe Accident Victims
React to Their Lot." *Journal of Personality and Social
Psychology* 35(1977):351-63.

Cassel, John, Ralph Patrick and David Jenkins. "Epidemiological
Analysis of the Health Implications of Culture Change: A
Conceptual Model." *Annals of the New York Academy of
Sciences* 84(1960):938-949.

Cassel, John and Herman A. Tyroler. "Epidemiological Studies of
Culture Change: I. Health Status and Recency of
Industrialization." *Archives of Environmental Health*
3(1961):25-33.

Cavan, Ruth S., Ernest W. Burgess, Robert J. Havighurst, and Herbert
Goldhamer. *Personal Adjustment in Old Age.* Chicago:
Science Research Associates, 1949.

Chanowitz, Benzion and Ellen Langer. "Knowing More (or Less)
Than You Can Show: Understanding Control Through the
Mindlessness-Mindfulness Distinction." In Garber, Judy, and
Martin E. P. Seligman, editors. *Human Helplessness: Theory
and Applications.* New York: Academic Press, 1980,
pp. 97-129.

Chodoff, Paul, Stanford B. Friedman, and David A. Hamburg. "Stress,
Defenses, and Coping Behavior: Observations in Parents of
Children With Malignant Disease." *American Journal of
Psychiatry* 120(1964):743-749.

Clark, Virginia A., Carol S. Aneshensel, Ralph R. Frerichs, and
Timothy M. Morgan. "Analysis of Effects of Sex and Age in
Response to Items on the CES-D Scale." *Psychiatry Research*
5(1981):171-181.

Cleary, Paul D. and Ronald Angel. "The Analysis of Relationships Involving Dichotomous Dependent Variables." *Journal of Health and Social Behavior* 25(1984):334-348.

Cobb, Sidney. "Social Support as a Moderator of Life Stress." *Psychosomatic Medicine* 38(1976):300-314.

Cobb, Sidney. "Social Support and Health Through the Life Course." In Riley, Matilda White, editor. *Aging From Birth to Death: Interdisciplinary Perspectives.* Boulder, Colorado: Westview Press, 1979.

Cockerham, William C., Kimberly Sharp, and Julie A. Wilcox. "Aging and Perceived Health Status." *Journal of Gerontology* 38(1983):349-355.

Cohen, Jacob and Patricia Cohen. *Applied Multiple Regression/Correlation Analysis for the Behavioral Sciences.* 2nd Edition. Hillsdale, N.J.: Lawrence Erlbaum, 1983.

Comer, Ronald and James D. Laird. "Choosing to Suffer as a Consequence of Expecting to Suffer: Why Do People Do It?" *Journal of Personality and Social Psychology* 32(1975):92-101.

Comstock, George W. and Knud J. Helsing. "Symptoms of Depression in Two Communities." *Psychological Medicine* 6(1976):551-563.

Comstock, George W. and Kay B. Partridge. "Church Attendance and Health." *Journal of Chronic Disease* 25(1972):665-672.

Comstock, George W. and James A. Tonascia. "Education and Mortality in Washington County, Maryland." *Journal of Health and Social Behavior* 18(1977):54-61.

Coyne, James C., Carolyn Aldwin, and Richard S. Lazarus. "Depression and Coping in Stressful Episodes." *Journal of Abnormal Psychology* 90(1981):439-447.

Croog, Sydney and Sol Levine. "Religious Identity and Response to Serious Illness: A Report on Heart Patients." *Social Science and Medicine* 6(1972):17-32.

Crystal, Stephen. *America's Old Age Crisis: Public Policy and the Two Worlds of Aging.* New York: Basic Books, 1982.

Cumming, E. and W.E. Henry. *Growing Old.* New York: Basic Books, 1961.

Cutler, Stephen J. "Membership in Different Types of Voluntary Associations and Psychological Well-Being." *The Gerontologist* 16(1976):335-339.

Dean, Alfred and Nan Lin. "The Stress-Buffering Role of Social Support." *Journal of Nervous and Mental Disease* 165(1977):403-417.

Deaux, Kay. "Sex: A Perspective on the Attribution Process." In Harvey, John H., William John Ickes, and Robert F. Kidd, editors. *New Directions in Attribution Research Vol.I.* Hillsdale, N.J.: Lawrence Erlbaum, 1976, pp. 335-352.

Dohrenwend, Barbara Snell, and Bruce P. Dohrenwend. *Stressful Life Events: Their Nature and Effects.* New York: John Wiley & Sons, 1974.

Dohrenwend, Bruce P. and Barbara Snell Dohrenwend. "Sex Differences and Psychiatric Disorders." *American Journal of Sociology* 81(1976):1447- 1454.

Dohrenwend, Bruce P. and Barbara Snell Dohrenwend. "Reply to Gove and Tudor's Comment on 'Sex Differences and Psychiatric Disorders.'" *American Journal of Sociology* 82(1977):1336-1345.

Douglas, Mary. *Natural Symbols: Explorations in Cosmology.* New York: Vintage Books, 1973.

Douglas, Mary. *Purity and Danger: An Analysis of the Concepts of Pollution and Taboo*. London: Routledge and Kegan Paul, 1966.

Durkheim, Emile. *The Division of Labor in Society*. Translated by George Simpson. New York: Free Press, 1964 (1933).

Durkheim, Emile. *Suicide: A Study in Sociology*. Translated by John A. Spaulding and George Simpson. New York: Free Press, 1951(1897).

Eaton, Joseph W. and Robert J. Weil. *Culture and Mental Disorders*. Glencoe, Illinois: Free Press, 1955.

Eaton, William W. and Larry G. Kessler. "Rates of Depression in a National Sample." *American Journal of Epidemiology* 114(1981):528-538.

Elshtain, Jean Bethke. *Public Man, Private Woman: Women in Social and Political Thought*. Princeton: Princeton University Press, 1981.

Faris, Robert E.L. and H. Warren Dunham. *Mental Disorders in Urban Areas: An Ecological Study of Schizophrenia and Other Psychoses*. Chicago: University of Chicago Press, 1967(1939).

Favazza, Armando R. "Modern Christian Healing of Mental Illness." *American Journal of Psychiatry* 139(1982):728-735.

Feifel, Herman and Allan B. Branscomb. "Who's Afraid of Death?" *Journal of Abnormal Psychology* 81(1973):282-288.

Feinberg, Stephen E. *The Analysis of Cross-Classified Categorical Data*. 2nd Edition. Cambridge, Mass.: MIT Press, 1980.

Ferraro, Kenneth F. "Self-Ratings of Health Among the Old and the Old-Old." *Journal of Health and Social Behavior* 21(1980):377-383.

Festinger, Leon, Henry W. Riecken and Stanley Schachter. *When Prophecy Fails: A Social and Psychological Study of a Modern Group that Predicted the Destruction of the World*. New York: Harper Torchbooks, 1964 [1956].

Fichter, Joseph. "The Profile of Catholic Religious Life." *American Journal of Sociology* 58(1952):145-149.

Fillenbaum, G.G. "Social Context and Self-Assessments of Health Among the Elderly." *Journal of Health and Social Behavior* 20(1979):45-51

Fischer, Claude S. *To Dwell Among Friends: Personal Networks in Town and City*. Chicago: University of Chicago Press, 1982.

Fischer, David Hackett. *Growing Old in America*. Oxford: Oxford University Press, 1978.

Folkman, Susan and Richard S. Lazarus. "An Analysis of Coping in a Middle-Aged Community Sample." *Journal of Health and Social Behavior* 21(1980):219-239.

Fowler, James W. *Stages of Faith: The Psychology of Human Development and the Quest for Meaning*. San Francisco: Harper & Row, 1981.

Freidson, Eliot. *Profession of Medicine: A Study of the Sociology of Applied Knowledge*. New York: Dodd, Mead, 1975.

Fukuyama, Yoshio. "The Major Dimensions of Church Membership." *Review of Religious Research* 2(1961):154-161.

Garber, Judy, Suzanne M. Miller, and Lyn Y. Abramson. "On the Distinction between Anxiety and Depression: Perceived Control, Certainty, and Probability of Goal Attainment." In Garber, Judy, and Martin E.P. Seligman, editors. *Human Helplessness: Theory and Applications*. New York: Academic Press, 1980, pp. 131-169.

Gardner, John W. and Joseph L. Lyon. "Cancer in Utah Mormon Men by Lay Priesthood Level." *American Journal of Epidemiology* 116(1982a):243- 257.

Gardner, John W. and Joseph L. Lyon. "Cancer in Utah Mormon Women by Church Activity Level." *American Journal of Epidemiology* 116(1982b):258-265.

Geertz, Clifford. *The Interpretation of Cultures.* New York: Basic Books, 1973.

Gilligan, Carol. *In a Different Voice.* Cambridge, Massachusetts: Harvard University Press, 1982.

Glock, Charles Y. and Rodney Stark. *Religion and Society in Tension.* Chicago: Rand McNally, 1965.

Glock, Charles Y. Benjamin B. Ringer and Earl R. Babbie. *To Comfort and To Challenge: A Dilemma of the Contemporary Church.* Berkeley: University of California Press, 1967.

Gore, Susan. "The Effect of Social Support in Moderating the Health Consequences of Unemployment". *Journal of Health and Social Behavior* 19(1978):157-165.

Gottlieb, Benjamin H., editor. *Social Networks and Social Support.* Beverly Hills: Sage Publications, 1981.

Gove, Walter F. and Jeannette F. Tudor. "Adult Sex Roles and Mental Illness." *American Journal of Sociology* 78(1973):812-835.

Gove, Walter F. and Jeannette F. Tudor. "Sex Differences in Mental Illness: A Comment on Dohrenwend and Dohrenwend." *American Journal of Sociology* 82(1977):1327-1345.

Graham, Thomas W. et al. "Frequency of Church Attendance and Blood Pressure Elevation." *Journal of Behavioral Medicine* 1(1978):37-43.

Granovetter, Mark S. "The Strength of Weak Ties." *American Journal of Sociology* 78(1973):1360-1380.

Gray, Robert M. and David O. Moberg. *The Church and the Older Person.* Grand Rapids: William B. Eerdmans, 1962.

Greeley, Andrew M. *Religion: A Secular Theory.* New York: Free Press, 1982.

Groen, J.J., K.B. Tijong, M. Koster, A.F. Willebrands, G. Verdonck, and M. Pierloot. "The Influence of Nutrition and Ways of Life on Blood Cholesterol and the Prevalence of Hypertension and Coronary Heart Disease Among Trappist and Benedictine Monks." *American Journal of Clinical Nutrition* 10(1962):456-470.

Gurin, Gerald, Joseph Veroff, and Sheila Feld. *Americans View Their Mental Health.* New York: Basic Books, 1960.

Gurland, Barry J. "The Comparative Frequency of Depression in Various Age Groups." *Journal of Gerontology* 31(1976):283-292.

Guttentag, Marcia, Susan Salasin, and Deborah Belle, editors. *The Mental Health of Women.* New York: Academic Press, 1980.

Hadaway, C. Kirk, Kirk W. Elifson, and David M. Petersen. "Religious Involvement and Drug Use among Urban Adolescents." *Journal for the Scientific Study of Religion* 23(1984):109-128.

Hannay, D.R. "Religion and Health." *Social Science and Medicine* 14A(1980):683-685.

Haug, Marie, Linda Liske Belgrave, and Brian Gratton. "Mental Health and the Elderly: Factors in Stability and Change Over Time." *Journal of Health and Social Behavior* 25(1984):100-115.

Heenan, Edward F. "Sociology of Religion and the Aged: The Empirical Lacunae." *Journal for the Scientific Study of Religion* 12(1972):171-176.

Heider, Fritz. *The Psychology of Interpersonal Relations*. New York: John Wiley, 1958.

Heisel, Marsel A. and Audrey O. Faulkner. "Religiosity in an Older Black Population." *The Gerontologist* 22(1982):354-358.

Helsing, Knud J., Moyses Szklo, and George W. Comstock. "Factors Associated with Mortality after Widowhood." *American Journal of Public Health* 71(1981):802-808.

Henderson, Scott, Paul Duncan-Jones, Helen McAuley, and Karen Ritchie. "The Patient's Primary Group." *British Journal of Psychiatry* 132(1978):74-86.

Herberg, Will. *Protestant-Catholic-Jew*. Garden City, New York: Anchor Books, 1960.

Hertz, Robert. *Death and the Right Hand*. Translated by Rodney and Claudia Needham. Glencoe, Illinois: Free Press, 1960 [1907, 1909].

Hinkle, Lawrence E. and Harold G. Wolff. "Ecologic Investigations of the Relationship between Illness, Life Experiences, and the Social Environment." *Annals of Internal Medicine* 49(1958):1373-1388.

Hochschild, Arlie Russell. "Disengagement Theory: A Critique and Proposal." *American Sociological Review* 40(1975):553-569.

Hollingshead, August B. and Frederick C. Redlich. *Social Class and Mental Illness: A Community Study*. New York: John Wiley & Sons, 1958.

Holmes, Thomas H. and R.H. Rahe. "The Social Readjustment Rating Scale." *Journal of Psychosomatic Research* 11(1967):213-218.

House, James S., Cynthia Robbins, and Helen L. Metzner. "The Association of Social Relationships and Activities with Mortality: Prospective Evidence From the Tecumseh Community Health Study." *American Journal of Epidemiology* 116(1982):123-140.

James, William. *The Varieties of Religious Experience.* New York: Doubleday, 1978 [1901-1902].

Jeffers, Frances C. and Adriaan Verwoerdt. "How the Old Face Death." In Ewald W. Busse and Eric Pfeiffer, editors. *Behavior and Adaptation in Late Life.* Boston: Little, Brown and Company, 1969, pp. 163-182.

Jenkins, C. David. "Psychologic and Social Precursors of Coronary Disease." *The New England Journal of Medicine* 284(1971):244-255, 307-317.

Jette, Alan M. and Laurence G. Branch. "The Framingham Disability Study: II. Physical Disability among the Aging." *American Journal of Public Health* 71(1981):1211-1216.

Jung, Carl. *Modern Man in Search of a Soul.* London: Kegan Paul, 1933.

Kalish, Richard A. and Ann I. Johnson. "Value Similarities and Differences in Three Generations of Women." *Journal of Marriage and the Family* 34(1972):49-54.

Kalish, Richard A. and David K. Reynolds. *Death and Ethnicity: A Psychocultural Study.* Los Angeles: University of Southern California Press, 1976.

Kanter, Rosabeth Moss. *Commitment and Community.* Cambridge, Mass.: Harvard University Press, 1972.

Kaplan, Berton H., John C. Cassel, and Susan Gore. "Social Support and Health." *Medical Care* 15 Supplement(1977):47-58.

Kaplan, George A. and Terry Camacho. "Perceived Health and Mortality: A Nine-Year Follow-Up of the Human Population Laboratory Cohort." *American Journal of Epidemiology* 117(1983):292-304.

Kasl, Stanislav V., Susan Gore, and Sidney Cobb. "The Experience of Losing a Job: Reported Changes in Health, Symptoms, and Illness Behavior." *Psychosomatic Medicine* 37(1975):106-122.

Katz, Alfred H. and Eugene I. Bender. *The Strength in Us: Self-Help Groups in the Modern World.* New York: New Viewpoints, 1976.

Katz, Sidney, Thomas Downs, Helen Cash, and Robert Grotz. "Progress in Development of the Index of Activities of Daily Living." *Gerontologist* Spring 1970, Part 1:20-30.

Kelley, Harold H. "Attribution Theory in Social Psychology." In D. Levine, editor. *Nebraska Symposium on Motivation* 15(1967):192-237, Lincoln: University of Nebraska Press.

Kelley, Harold H. "Moral Evaluation." *American Psychologist* 26(1971):293-300.

Kelsey, Morton T. *Healing and Christianity.* New York: Harper and Row, 1973.

Kessler, Ronald C. and James A. McRae. "Trends in the Relationship Between Sex and Psychological Distress, 1957-1976." *American Sociological Review* 46(1981):443-452.

Kleinbaum, David G. and Lawrence L. Kupper. *Applied Regression Analysis and Other Multivariable Methods.* North Scituate, Mass.: Duxbury Press, 1978.

Kohn, Melvin. "Class, Family, and Schizophrenia." *Social Forces* 50(1972):295-304.

Komarovsky, Mirra. *Blue-Collar Marriage*. New York: Random House, 1962.

Kubler-Ross, Elizabeth. *On Death and Dying*. New York: MacMillan, 1969.

Lakoff, George and Mark Johnson. *Metaphors We Live By*. Chicago: University of Chicago Press, 1980.

Langer, Ellen J. *The Psychology of Control*. Beverly Hills: Sage Publications, 1983.

Langlie, Jean K. "Social Networks, Health Beliefs, and Preventive Health Behavior." *Journal of Health and Social Behavior* 18(1977):244-260.

LaRue, Asenath, Lew Bank, Lissy Jarvik, and Monte Hetland. "Health in Old Age: How do Physicians' Ratings and Self-Ratings Compare?" *Journal of Gerontology* 34(1979):687-691.

LaRocco, James M., James S. House, and John R. French. "Social Support, Occupational Stress, and Health." *Journal of Health and Social Behavior* 21(1980):202-218.

Laumann, Edward O. *Bonds of Pluralism: The Form and Substance of Urban Social Networks*. New York: John Wiley, 1973.

Lazarus, R.S., and R. Launier. "Stress-Related Transactions Between Person and Environment." In L.A. Pervin and M. Lewis, editors. *Perspectives in Interactional Psychology*. New York: Plenum, 1978.

Lazerwitz, Bernard. "A Comparison of Major United States Religious Groups." *American Statistical Association Journal* 56(1961):568-579.

Lefcourt, Herbert M. "Personality and Locus of Control." In Garber, Judy and Martin E.P. Seligman, editors. *Human Helplessness: Theory and Applications*. New York: Academic Press, 1980, pp. 245-260.

Leighton, Dorothea et al. *The Character of Danger Vol.III*. New York: Basic Books, 1963.

Lenski, Gerhard. "Social Correlates of Religious Interest." *American Sociological Review* 18(1953):533-544.

Lerner, M.J. "The Desire for Justice and Reactions to Victims." In J. Macaulay and L. Berkowitz, editors. *Altruism and Helping Behavior*. New York: Academic Press, 1970.

Lester, David. "Experimental and Correlational Studies of the Fear of Death." *Psychological Bulletin* 67(1967):27-36.

Lewis, C.S. *The Problem of Pain*. New York: MacMillan Publishing Co., 1962.

Lieberman, Morton A. and Annie Siranne Coplan. "Distance From Death as a Variable in the Study of Aging." *Developmental Psychology* 2(1970):71-84.

Liem, Ramsay and Joan Liem. "Social Class and Mental Illness Reconsidered: The Role of Economic Stress and Social Support." *Journal of Health and Social Behavior* 19(1978):139-156.

Lindenthal, Jacob J., Jerome K. Myers, Max P. Pepper, and Maxine S. Stern. "Mental Status and Religious Behavior." *Journal for the Scientific Study of Religion* 9(1970):143-149.

Lowenthal, Marjorie Fisk and Clayton Haven. "Interaction and Adaptation: Intimacy as a Critical Variable." *American Sociological Review* 33(1968):20-30.

Luckmann, Thomas. *The Invisible Religion*. London: Macmillan, 1967.

McCready, William C. and Andrew M. Greeley. *The Ultimate Values of the American Population.* Beverly Hills: Sage Publications, 1976.

McGuire, Meredith. *Pentecostal Catholics: Power, Charisma, and Order in a Religious Movement.* Philadelphia: Temple University Press, 1982.

McMordie, William R. "Religiosity and Fear of Death." *Psychological Reports* 49(1981):921-922.

Maddox, George L. "Some Correlates of Difference in Self-Assessment of Health Status Among the Elderly." *Journal of Gerontology* 17(1962):180-185.

Maddox, George L. and Elizabeth B. Douglass. "Self-Assessment of Health: A Longitudinal Study of Elderly Subjects." *Journal of Health and Social Behavior* 14(1973):87-93.

Malinowski, B. *Magic, Science, and Religion.* Boston, 1948.

Maranell, Gary M. *Responses to Religion: Studies in the Social Psychology of Religious Belief.* Lawrence, Kansas: The University Press of Kansas, 1974.

Martin, David and Lawrence S. Wrightsman. "The Relationship Between Religious Behavior and Concern About Death." *The Journal of Social Psychology* 65(1965):317-323.

Masuda, Minoru and Thomas H. Holmes. "Life Events: Perceptions and Frequencies." *Psychosomatic Medicine* 40(1978):236-261.

Mather, Cotton. *Addresses to Old Men and Young Men and Little Children.* Boston, 1690.

Mather, Increase. *The Dignity and Duty of Aged Servants.* Boston, 1716.

Maves, Paul B. "Aging, Religion, and the Church." In Clark Tibbits, editor. *Handbook of Social Gerontology.* Chicago: University of Chicago Press, 1960, pp. 698-749.

Mechanic, David. "Development of Psychological Distress Among Young Adults." *Archives of General Psychiatry* 36(1979):1233-1239.

Medalie, Jack H., Harold A. Kahn, Henry N. Neufeld, Egon Riss, and Uri Goldbourt. "Five-Year Myocardial Infarction Incidence-II. Association of Single Variables to Age and Birthplace." *Journal of Chronic Disease* 26(1973):329-349.

Mindel, Charles H. and C. Edwin Vaughan. "A Multidimensional Approach to Religiosity and Disengagement." *Journal of Gerontology* 33(1978):103-108.

Mitchell, J.C., editor. *Social Networks and Urban Situations.* Manchester: Manchester University Press, 1969.

Moberg, David O. "Religion in Old Age." *Geriatrics* (1965):977-982.

Morris, P.A. "Effect of Pilgrimage on Anxiety, Depression, and Religious Attitude." *Psychological Medicine* 12(1982):291-294.

Mossey, Jana M. and Evelyn Shapiro. "Self-Rated Health: A Predictor of Mortality Among the Elderly." *American Journal of Public Health* 72(1982):800-808.

Mueller, Daniel P. "Social Networks: A Promising Direction for Research on the Relationship of the Social Environment to Psychiatric Disorder." *Social Science and Medicine* 14A(1980):147-161.

Myers, Jerome K., Jacob J. Lindenthal, and Max P. Pepper. "Life Events, Social Integration, and Psychiatric Symptomatology." *Journal of Health and Social Behavior* 16(1975):421-427.

Nagi, Saad Z. "An Epidemiology of Disability among Adults in the United States." *Milbank Memorial Fund Quarterly Health and Society* 54(1976):439-467.

Nathanson, Constance A. "Illness and the Feminine Role: A Theoretical Review." *Social Science and Medicine* 9(1975):57-62.

Ness, Robert C. "The Impact of Indigenous Healing Activity: An Empirical Study of Two Fundamentalist Churches." *Social Science and Medicine* 14B(1980):167-180.

Nuckolls, Katherine B., John Cassel, and Berton H. Kaplan. "Psychosocial Assets, Life Crisis, and the Prognosis of Pregnancy." *American Journal of Epidemiology* 95(1972):431-441.

Orbach, Harold L. "Aging and Religion: A Study of Church Attendance in the Detroit Metropolitan Area." *Geriatrics* 16(1961):530-540.

Orvis, Bruce R., Harold H. Kelley, and Deborah Butler. "Attributional Conflict in Young Couples." In John H. Harvey, William John Ickes, Robert F. Kidd, editors. *New Directions in Attribution Research*. Hillsdale, N.J.: Lawrence Erlbaum Associates, 1976, pp. 353-386.

Otto, Rudolf. *The Idea of the Holy*. Translated by John W. Harvey. London: Oxford University Press, 1978 [1917].

Palmore, Erdman. "The Sociological Aspects of Aging." In Ewald W. Busse and Eric Pfeiffer, editors. *Behavior and Adaptation in Late Life*. Boston: Little, Brown and Company, 1969, pp. 33-70.

Parkes, C. Murray, B. Benjamin, and R.G. Fitzgerald. "Broken Heart: A Statistical Study of Increased Mortality Among Widowers." *British Medical Journal* 1(1969):740-743.

Pattison, E. Mansell et al. "A Psychosocial Kinship Model for Family Therapy." *American Journal of Psychiatry* 132(1975):1246-1251.

Paykel, Eugene, Jerome K. Myers, Marcia Dienelt, Gerald Klerman, Jacob J. Lindenthal, and Max Pepper. "Life Events and Depression: A Controlled Study." *Archives of General Psychiatry* 21(1969):753-760.

Pearlin, Leonard I. and Carmi Schooler. "The Structure of Coping." *Journal of Health and Social Behavior* 19(1978):2-21.

Princeton Religion Research Center. *Religion in America 1982.* Princeton, 1982.

Proudfoot, Wayne and Phillip Shaver. "Attribution Theory and the Psychology of Religion." *Journal for the Scientific Study of Religion* 14(1975):317-330.

Radcliffe-Brown, A.R. *Structure and Function in Primitive Society.* New York: Free Press, 1965 [1952].

Radloff, Lenore. "Sex Differences in Depression: The Effects of Occupation and Marital Status." *Sex Roles* 1(1975):249-265.

Radloff, Lenore. "The CES-D Scale: A Self-Report Depression Scale for Research in the General Population." *Applied Psychological Measurement* 1(1977):385-401.

Radloff, Lenore. "Risk Factors for Depression: What Do We Learn From Them?" In Guttentag, Marcia, Susan Salasin, and Deborah Belle, editors. *The Mental Health of Women.* New York: Academic Press, 1980.

Rainwater, Lee. "The Problem of Lower-Class Culture and Poverty-War Strategy." In Daniel P. Moynihan, editor. *On Understanding Poverty.* New York: Basic Books, 1969, pp. 229-259.

Reed, Dwayne, Daniel McGee, and Katsuhiko Yano. "Psychosocial Processes and General Susceptibility to Chronic Disease." *American Journal of Epidemiology* 119(1984):356-370.

Riley, Matilda White, and Anne Foner. *Aging and Society Vol.I: An Inventory of Research Findings.* New York: Russell Sage, 1968.

Rizley, Ross. "Depression and Distortion in the Attribution of Causality." *Journal of Abnormal Psychology* 87(1978):32-48.

Roberts, Bertram H. and Jerome K. Myers. "Religion, National Origin, Immigration, and Mental Illness." *American Journal of Psychiatry* 110(1954):759-764.

Rosaldo, M.Z. "The Use and Abuse of Anthropology: Reflections on Feminism and Cross-Cultural Understanding." *Signs: Journal of Women in Culture and Society* 5(1980):389-417.

Rosow, Irving. *Socialization to Old Age.* Berkeley: University of California Press, 1974.

Rosow, Irving and Naomi Breslau. "A Guttman Health Scale for the Aged." *Journal of Gerontology* 21(1966):556-559.

Rotter, J.B. "Generalized Expectancies for Internal versus External Control of Reinforcement." *Psychological Monographs* 80(1966):1-28.

Rubin, Zick and Letitia Anne Peplau. "Who Believes in a Just World?" *Journal of Social Issues* 31(1975):65-89.

Sargant, William. "The Physiology of Faith." *British Journal of Psychiatry* 115(1969):505-518.

Scarf, Maggie. *Unfinished Business: Pressure Points in the Lives of Women.* New York: Ballantine, 1980.

Schulz, James H. *The Economics of Aging*. 2nd edition. Belmont, California: Wadsworth Publishing Co., 1980.

Scotch, Norman, A. "Sociocultural Factors in the Epidemiology of Zulu Hypertension." *American Journal of Public Health* 53(1963):1205-1213.

Seligman, Martin E.P. *Helplessness: On Depression, Development, and Death*. San Francisco: W.H.Freeman, 1975.

Silver, Roxane L. and Camille B. Wortman. "Coping with Undesirable Life Events." In Garber, Judy and Martin E.P. Seligman, editors. *Human Helplessness: Theory and Applications*. New York: Academic Press, 1980, pp. 279-340.

Snow, David A. and Richard Machalek. "On the Presumed Fragility of Unconventional Beliefs." *Journal for the Scientific Study of Religion* 21(1982):15-26.

Srole, Leo, Thomas S. Langer, Stanley Michael, Marvin Opler, and Thomas A.C. Rennie. *Mental Health in the Metropolis: The Midtown Manhattan Study*. New York: McGraw-Hill, 1962.

Stark, Rodney. "Age and Faith: A Changing Outlook or an Old Process?" *Sociological Analysis* 29(1968):1-10.

Steinitz, Lucy Y. "Religiosity, Well-Being, and Weltanschauung Among the Elderly." *Journal for the Scientific Study of Religion* 19(1980):60-67.

Stoller, Eleanor Palo. "Self-Assessments of Health by the Elderly: The Impact of Informal Assistance." *Journal of Health and Social Behavior* 25(1984):260-270.

Swenson, Wendell M. "Attitudes Toward Death in an Aged Population." *Journal of Gerontology* 16(1961):49-52.

Templer, Donald I. "Death Anxiety in Religiously Very Involved Persons." *Psychological Reports* 31(1972):361-362.

Templer, Donald I. and Elsie Dotson. "Religious Correlates of Death Anxiety." *Psychological Reports* 26(1970):895-897.

Tessler, Richard and David Mechanic. "Psychological Distress and Perceived Health Status." *Journal of Health and Social Behavior* 19(1978):254-262.

Thoits, Peggy A. "Conceptual, Methodological, and Theoretical Problems in Studying Social Support as a Buffer Against Life Stress." *Journal of Health and Social Behavior* 23(1982):145-159.

Turner, R. Jay. "Social Support as a Contingency in Psychological Well-Being." *Journal of Health and Social Behavior* 22(1981):357-367.

Turner, Victor. *The Ritual Process: Structure and Anti-Structure.* Ithaca: Cornell University Press, 1969.

Tyroler, H.A. and John Cassel. "Health Consequences of Culture Change-II: The Effect of Urbanization on Coronary Heart Mortality in Rural Residents." *Journal of Chronic Disease* 17(1964):167-177.

Ulbrich, Holley and Myles Wallace. "Women's Work Force Status and Church Attendance." *Journal for the Scientific Study of Religion* 23(1984):341-350.

U. S. Department of Commerce, Bureau of the Census. *Statistical Abstract of the United States 100th edition.* Washington, D.C.: 1979.

Van Gennep, Arnold. *The Rites of Passage.* Translated by Monika Vizedom and Gabrielle L. Caffee. Chicago: University of Chicago Press, 1960 [1908].

Vaux, Kenneth L. *This Mortal Coil: The Meaning of Health and Disease.* San Francisco: Harper & Row, 1978.

Vaux, Kenneth L. *Health and Medicine in the Reformed Tradition: Promise, Providence and Care.* New York: Crossroads, 1984.

Walster, Elaine. "Assignment of Responsibility for an Accident." *Journal of Personality and Social Psychology* 3(1966):73-79.

Weber, Max. *Economy and Society Vols. I and II.* Edited by Guenther Roth and Claus Wittich. Berkeley: University of California Press, 1978.

Weber, Max. *The Sociology of Religion.* Translated by Ephraim Fischoff. Boston: Beacon Press, 1964 [1922].

Weiner, Bernard. *Theories of Motivation: From Mechanism to Cognition.* Chicago: Rand McNally College Publishing Co., 1972.

Weiss, Robert S. "The Fund of Sociability." *Trans-Action* July/August 1969:36-43.

Weissman, Myrna K. and Jerome K. Myers. "Depression in the Elderly: Research Directions in Psychopathology, Epidemiology, and Treatment." *Journal of Geriatric Psychiatry* 12(1979):187-201.

Wellman, Barry. "Applying Network Analysis to the Study of Support." In Benjamin H. Gottlieb, editor. *Social Networks and Social Support.* Beverly Hills: Sage Publications, 1981, pp. 171-200.

Westbrook, Mary T. and Linda L. Viney. "Age and Sex Differences in Patients' Reactions to Illness." *Journal of Health and Social Behavior* 24(1983):313-324.

Wheaton, Blair. "The Sociogenesis of Psychological Disorder: Reexamining the Causal Issues with Longitudinal Data." *American Sociological Review* 43(1978):383-403.

Wheaton, Blair. "The Sociogenesis of Psychological Disorder: An Attributional Theory." *Journal of Health and Social Behavior* 21(1980):100-124.

Wheaton, Blair. "Stress, Personal Coping Resources, and Psychiatric Symptoms: An Investigation of Interactive Models." *Journal of Health and Social Behavior* 24(1983):208-229.

Wicklund, Robert A. "Objective Self-Awareness." in L. Berkowitz, editor. *Advances in Experimental Social Psychology Vol.8.* New York: Academic Press, 1975.

Williams, Robert L. and Spurgeon Cole. "Religiosity, Generalized Anxiety, and Apprehension Concerning Death." *Journal of Social Psychology* 75(1968):111-117.

Wingard, Deborah. "The Sex Differential in Mortality Rates: Demographic and Behavioral Factors." *American Journal of Epidemiology* 115(1982):205-16.

Wingrove, C. Ray and Jon P. Alston. "Cohort Analysis of Church Attendance, 1939-69." *Social Forces* 53(1974):324-331.

Wortman, Camille and Jack W. Brehm. "Responses to Uncontrollable Outcomes: An Integration of Reactance Theory and the Learned Helplessness Model." In L. Berkowitz, editor. *Advances in Experimental Social Psychology* Vol.8(1975):277-336.

Wuthnow, Robert, Kevin Christiano, and John Kuzlowski. "Religion and Bereavement: A Conceptual Framework." *Journal for the Scientific Study of Religion* 19(1980):408-422.

Wynder, Ernest L., Frank R. Lemon, and Irwin J. Bross. "Cancer and Coronary Artery Disease Among Seventh-Day Adventists." *Cancer* 12(1959):1016-1028.

Zuckerman, Diana M., Stanislav V. Kasl, and Adrian M. Ostfeld. "Psychosocial Predictors of Mortality Among the Elderly Poor: The Role of Religion, Well-Being, and Social Contacts." *American Journal of Epidemiology* 119(1984):410-423.

Appendix A. Center for Epidemiologic Studies Depression Scale

	Rarely or none of the time	Some of the time	Much of the time	Most or all of the time
1. I was bothered by things that ususally don't bother me.	1	2	3	4
2. I did not feel like eating; my appetite was poor	1	2	3	4
3. I felt that I could not shake off the blues.	1	2	3	4
4. I felt that I was just as good as other people.	4	3	2	1
5. I had trouble keeping my mind on what I was doing.	1	2	3	4
6. I felt depressed.	1	2	3	4
7. I felt that everything I did was an effort.	1	2	3	4
8. I felt hopeful about the future.	4	3	2	1
9. I thought my life had been a failure.	1	2	3	4
10. I felt fearful.	1	2	3	4
11. My sleep was restless.	1	2	3	4
12. I was happy.	4	3	2	1
13. It seemed that I talked less than usual.	1	2	3	4
14. I felt lonely.	1	2	3	4
15. People were unfriendly.	1	2	3	4
16. I enjoyed life.	4	3	2	1
17. I had crying spells.	1	2	3	4
18. I felt sad.	1	2	3	4
19. I felt that people disliked me.	1	2	3	4
20. I could not get going.	1	2	3	4

Appendix B. Observed frequencies for men's religious involvement, social networks, meaning, and fatalism

Attend	Comfort	Network	Meaning	Fatalism	KNOW None/Few IDENTITY			KNOW Many/All IDENTITY		
					Deeply	Fairly	Not	Deeply	Fairly	Not
Never	Much	0-8	Hopeful	Helpless	7	3	2	2	3	0
				Not	2	2	4	1	1	0
			Not	Helpless	6	2	1	1	3	0
				Not	5	6	2	0	1	0
		9+	Hopeful	Helpless	3	5	0	1	3	0
				Not	1	2	2	4	1	0
			Not	Helpless	7	3	1	2	1	0
				Not	4	3	1	1	2	0
	Little	0-8	Hopeful	Helpless	0	3	5	1	0	0
				Not	0	9	6	0	0	0
			Not	Helpless	3	5	14	0	0	1
				Not	0	9	23	0	2	2
		9+	Hopeful	Helpless	1	5	2	0	2	0
				Not	0	5	6	0	1	0
			Not	Helpless	0	5	2	0	1	0
				Not	1	7	6	0	0	3
Rarely	Much	0-8	Hopeful	Helpless	3	3	0	1	3	2
				Not	2	4	0	0	4	0
			Not	Helpless	1	7	2	1	2	0
				Not	1	8	0	1	4	1
		9+	Hopeful	Helpless	3	4	1	3	1	3
				Not	3	3	5	5	10	1
			Not	Helpless	6	5	0	2	3	0
				Not	11	10	0	7	3	2
	Little	0-8	Hopeful	Helpless	1	2	1	1	2	0
				Not	0	5	4	0	5	2
			Not	Helpless	0	8	10	0	1	1
				Not	0	5	7	1	2	5
		9+	Hopeful	Helpless	0	8	4	1	2	2
				Not	2	7	5	1	8	3
			Not	Helpless	1	5	3	0	2	3
				Not	1	5	6	2	5	7
Often	Much	0-8	Hopeful	Helpless	7	8	0	5	12	1
				Not	3	4	0	7	13	1
			Not	Helpless	4	1	2	12	8	0
				Not	7	6	0	10	7	0
		9+	Hopeful	Helpless	3	6	0	26	24	1
				Not	2	15	1	32	37	0
			Not	Helpless	4	4	0	23	8	1
				Not	11	9	0	46	26	4
	Little	0-8	Hopeful	Helpless	0	1	2	1	5	4
				Not	1	2	2	0	5	3
			Not	Helpless	0	2	1	3	0	5
				Not	0	6	2	0	4	2
		9+	Hopeful	Helpless	1	4	0	0	4	1
				Not	0	6	1	2	12	4
			Not	Helpless	0	2	1	2	5	3
				Not	3	4	3	1	8	6

Appendix B. Observed frequencies for women's religious involvement, social networks, meaning, and fatalism

Attend	Comfort	Network	Meaning	Fatalism	KNOW None/Few IDENTITY			KNOW Many/All IDENTITY		
					Deeply	Fairly	Not	Deeply	Fairly	Not
Never	Much	0-8	Hopeful	Helpless	10	8	2	6	5	0
				Not	11	8	1	2	5	0
			Not	Helpless	14	9	4	5	2	1
				Not	14	9	1	3	2	0
		9+	Hopeful	Helpless	8	8	2	4	3	0
				Not	9	10	3	4	2	0
			Not	Helpless	7	3	1	5	2	0
				Not	9	6	2	1	2	0
	Little	0-8	Hopeful	Helpless	0	7	2	0	0	0
				Not	2	8	5	0	0	0
			Not	Helpless	4	8	10	2	2	0
				Not	1	10	8	0	0	3
		9+	Hopeful	Helpless	1	3	4	0	4	1
				Not	1	4	5	0	0	1
			Not	Helpless	1	6	4	0	2	1
				Not	0	7	3	0	0	0
Rarely	Much	0-8	Hopeful	Helpless	4	7	1	5	3	1
				Not	3	9	0	6	9	0
			Not	Helpless	18	3	0	1	3	0
				Not	10	6	0	7	8	0
		9+	Hopeful	Helpless	5	7	1	4	11	0
				Not	3	8	0	2	8	1
			Not	Helpless	4	1	2	6	7	0
				Not	12	10	1	9	6	0
	Little	0-8	Hopeful	Helpless	0	0	1	0	1	1
				Not	0	7	4	0	2	1
			Not	Helpless	0	5	2	0	1	1
				Not	2	12	3	0	2	1
		9+	Hopeful	Helpless	0	2	4	0	4	2
				Not	1	2	3	0	4	6
			Not	Helpless	0	6	2	0	6	2
				Not	0	3	1	1	4	2
Often	Much	0-8	Hopeful	Helpless	16	12	1	35	19	0
				Not	9	18	2	25	18	1
			Not	Helpless	14	14	5	26	14	0
				Not	8	12	1	31	21	2
		9+	Hopeful	Helpless	9	12	1	54	47	2
				Not	15	18	0	42	45	1
			Not	Helpless	11	8	0	30	15	0
				Not	19	10	1	83	23	0
	Little	0-8	Hopeful	Helpless	1	4	2	0	5	2
				Not	2	2	0	1	4	3
			Not	Helpless	1	2	2	0	6	0
				Not	2	6	2	0	5	0
		9+	Hopeful	Helpless	0	2	0	0	11	2
				Not	0	5	1	1	8	1
			Not	Helpless	0	1	0	0	2	1
				Not	0	4	0	1	6	0

Name Index

Subject Index